Henry Gradle

Bacteria and the Germ Theory of Disease

Henry Gradle

Bacteria and the Germ Theory of Disease

ISBN/EAN: 9783742806055

Manufactured in Europe, USA, Canada, Australia, Japa

Cover: Foto ©Lupo / pixelio.de

Manufactured and distributed by brebook publishing software
(www.brebook.com)

Henry Gradle

Bacteria and the Germ Theory of Disease

BACTERIA

AND

THE GERM THEORY OF DISEASE.

EIGHT LECTURES DELIVERED AT THE

CHICAGO MEDICAL COLLEGE,

BY

Dr. H. GRADLE,

PROF. OF PHYSIOLOGY, CHICAGO MEDICAL COLLEGE; OCULIST TO THE
MICHAEL REESE HOSPITAL.

CHICAGO:
W. T. KEENER, 96 WASHINGTON STREET.
1883.

CONTENTS.

LECTURE I.

LECTURE II.

LECTURE III.

LECTURE IV.

LECTURE V.

LECTURE VI.

LECTURE VII.

LECTURE VIII.

THE GERM-THEORY OF DISEASE.

LECTURE I.

In no department of medicine is there a greater
separation between our present knowledge and the
views of our ancestors, than in Ætiology. In most
other branches of medical science we stand upon the
shoulders of those who preceded us. The therapeutic
practice of to-day, however superior to that of the
last century, has been evolved so gradually, has
passed through such a continuous transition, that it
would be difficult to point out any one period as the
beginning of a new epoch. But the knowledge of the
causes of disease is an acquisition of the most recent
times, is the work only of the present generation. The
vague references of former physicians to impurities of
the blood, chemical dyscrasia, a genius epidemicus, and

the exaggerated belief in that omnipotent bug-bear—
cold—we can but regard as speculations without basis.
Without underrating the earnest work done by medical
men of a former period, it is evident that the causes of
diseases, with the exception of some of the more patent
instances, escaped them. It is only within the last twenty
years, or less, that evidence is accumulating showing that
many ailments to which flesh is heir, are due to the
invasion of the organism by microscopic parasites or
their germs.   Daily, almost, new facts are discovered,
which substantiate more and more this *germ theory of
disease.* In the light of the germ theory, diseases are
to be considered as *a struggle between the organism and
the parasites invading it.* As far as the germ theory is
applicable, it eliminates the factor "accident" from the
consideration of disease, and assigns disease a place in
the Darwinian programme of nature.

In the modern conception disease is a disturbance of
the normal play of some one, or different parts of the
organism, the reaction to an unaccustomed influence.
According to the germ theory, the foreign influence producing this disturbance, is in very many instances the
existence of foreign microscopic beings in the interior
of the animal body, and the number of diseases of which
the germ theory reveals the origin, is constantly aug-
menting.

Yet the germ theory meets still with much opposition
and, what is worse, indifference, and nowhere more than
in this country.   Much of this opposition is due to—
ignorance. I would account for this in the following
way: There is but little original work published on this
topic in the English language, especially in this country.
Although foreign discoveries soon find their way into
our journals, they appear, as a rule, in the form of an

abstract, without much description of the methods used in obtaining the results. But the fruits of experimental sciences can only be well appreciated by him who knows how they were obtained. If we cannot critically examine the methods, we are at a loss in assigning the proper value to the conclusions, so that the most conscientious work may be received with distrust, because we are unprepared for its results, while the illogical conclusions of another author are sometimes implicitly accepted, because they agree with prior notions. Certainly no other experimental science can offer greater contrasts than research on the germ theory between thorough investigation on the one hand, and almost valueless work on the other. With some familiarity, however, with the literature, one learns to distinguish readily between some slipshod observations, and hasty conclusions therefrom, and the more reliable results obtained by methods which equal in accuracy those employed in physical sciences.

If we were to drop our acquired medical notions, and were to approach the study of disease from the standpoint of the modern naturalist, the germ theory would present itself in a more attractive light. Throughout nature every species of living beings struggles for its existence with all other beings with which it comes in immediate contact. In numerous instances this struggle amounts to the preying of a smaller species upon the body of larger creatures, the former deriving from the organism of their host their means of subsistence.

Throughout the animal and the vegetable kingdoms, parasitism is of common occurrence. Often the host carries but a single invader, but as the discrepancy

between the size of the parasite and the organism
harboring it, increases, the number of the intruders is
also apt to enlarge. The greater the difference in the
dimensions of the contending beings, and the wider
they are apart in the botanical or zoological scale, the
more desperate does the struggle become. If the host
cannot oppose a resistance to the attack of the
invaders, cannot dislodge them in time, he is doomed
to succumb. No botanist would be at a loss to illustrate this occurrence by reference to numerous
instances in the vegetable kingdom, the most frequent
examples being a struggle between the higher plants
and fungi. Indeed it is claimed that all diseases of
plants are of parasitic origin. The role of the lower
organism is too plain in such cases to admit of a
doubt, while its size renders the investigation comparatively simple.

The parasitic existence of lower animals in the
bodies of higher beings is also a common observation.
But unless these parasites are present in large numbers they do not usually compromise the health of
their host to any great extent, as an instance of which
I might mention intestinal worms. It is only when
we observe beings of such microscopic dimensions and
consequent multitude in numbers as the trichina
spiralis, or the filaria, found in the blood of chyluria,
that we see health and life seriously menaced by the
invasion of animal parasites. Much more numerous,
however, are diseases traceable to the development of
lower plants in the interior of animal bodies. Instances of this occurrence can be found in all animals
down to insects and worms. In proof of this statement I cannot do better than dwell at some length
upon one of the best studied examples of a parasitic

disease in lower animals—viz: the pebrine of the silk-worm.

This disease occurs in epidemics in silk-raising districts, sometimes to such an extent as almost to annihilate that industry. The caterpillars attacked by it show black spots on their skin, lose their appetite and die. In the blood and all the tissues of the worm small oval granules were observed by various investigators. Although these granules were recognized as a species of the lowest fungi, their relation to the disease was not established until Pasteur proved them to be the cause. In simple but conclusive experiments he showed that the disease could be produced in healthy specimens by feeding them on material containing these granules, or by inoculating them from a wound. On the basis of positive observations he explained thus the spreading of the epidemic. He further showed that the butterfly transmits the disease to its offspring, in case it survives up to the act of copulation. For the parasitic growth can be found in the egg, if either male or female be tainted with the disease. Although Pasteur did not succeed in finding any means of arresting the disease in the individual animal, he taught the silk raisers how to check the epidemic. The copulating insects which at this stage of their existence are doomed to die any way, are examined microscopically, and the eggs of all diseased butterflies are destroyed. The healthy eggs raised in a disinfected locality reproduce a healthy stock. No more eloquent proof can be given of the importance of Pasteur's work than a statistical report of the silk industry of France. While the silk crop of 1853 amounted to 26,000,000 kilograms, it had fallen gradually in consequence of the disease to 4,000,000 kilo-

grams in 1865. Since the application of the scientific
triumphs achieved by Pasteur, the disease has been
practically exterminated and the crops have risen
again to their former standard. So much for the
practical application of the germ theory to a disease
of lower animals! Of course it might be said, and it
has been said, that research on lower animals can
throw no light on human pathology, but do such
gratuitous assertions, bred of ignorance and prejudice,
deserve serious consideration?

As an instance of vegetable parasites found in diseases of the higher animals and man, I need but
refer to certain affections of the skin. It is now
generally admitted that various skin diseases are due
to the growth of different fungi on the affected spot.
But as regards such parasites living only on the surface of the body, you will find ample information in
any of the text-books on skin diseases. Hence I can
pass at once to the description of those parasites
which enter into the interior of the system, and
which have of late attracted most attention, as the
presumptive cause of most general diseases, viz.:
bacteria.

This species of microscopic beings consists of uni-
cellular organisms, the smallest representatives of ani-
mated nature. Certain peculiarities in the nutrition
and mode of reproduction, upon which we shall dwell
later, characterize them as plants. They are commonly
classed as the lowest forms of fungi. In fact, the
Germans call them "Spaltpilze," *dividing fungi* (also
Schizomycetæ or Schistomycetæ). If we include among
the fungi all plants which lack chlorophyll, or some
equivalent pigment, the bacteria belong to this class.
But morphologically they differ from the true fungi

in consisting of single short cells, not ramifying into a mycelium. In their form, on the other hand, they resemble the algæ, but differ again from them in not containing chlorophyll. However, leaving to botanists the mooted question whether the bacteria are to rank with one or the other group of plants, or whether they constitute a genus by themselves, we will proceed to study their mode of life. It will be the better plan to describe in the first place the bacteria which we encounter outside of the animal body.

The earliest use of the microscope in the hands of Leeuwenhoek showed that these minute organisms abound wherever processes of decomposition or putrefaction occur. A drop of water from a stagnant pool, a fragment of an animal cadaver, or of vegetable refuse, all teem with microscopic life. We need not concern ourselves at present with the infusorial animals or the algæ likely to be encountered there as well; for while these forms frequently inhabit the same soil in common with bacteria, they are irrelevant to our topic. Appearing in the form of minute granules and variously shaped rods, the bacteria tax the power of the microscope for their sharp definition. The larger rods, especially when closely grouped, can be seen with a power of 100 to 200 diameters, while the finer granules require an amplification of 400 times or more for their mere detection. Wherever dead animal or vegetable material is left in a moist state, bacteria make their appearance. No putrefaction or rotting occurs in which their presence cannot be shown. In the words of the French dramatist Dumas: "They are the agents of corruption in nature."

That these apparently structureless rods and granules are living beings is proven by their power of multiplication. The best, and sometimes the only criterion of life in the case of the lowest organisms is the capability of reproducing their kind under proper conditions. With sufficient patience we can watch a bacterium growing in size and ultimately dividing into two or more fragments similar in form, but of course smaller, than the parent. We can demonstrate their multiplication even in a more simple manner, without such painstaking observations; for if a single one of these organisms, or at least the smallest practical number, be introduced into a fluid, like meat infusion, in which they find nourishment, they will speedily multiply. Though this fluid may have been clear as crystal originally, it becomes turbid from the presence of myriads of bacteria.

Before inquiring as to the relation of bacteria to putrefaction, it will be well to give a precise definition of the latter term. Every day experience shows us that, while inorganic substances are chemically stable, dead organic material left to itself will gradually change in appearance,—in other words, it decomposes. As a rule it loses its consistency, becomes softer, and ultimately liquefies. The decomposition is furthermore indicated by a disagreeable odor. In fact, popularly the nose is the judge of decomposition, and we seldom think of rottenness without smell. But the smell varies with the nature · of the material. The chemical substances to which it is due are ammonia, sulphuretted hydrogen, sometimes phosphoretted hydrogen, various volatile fatty acids, like butyric, valerianic, ʹcaprylic, and other acids, besides traces of many other organic compounds. Further examination shows that putrefaction consists of a very complicated series of chemical changes.

From the fact that fresh animal and vegetable tissues are mixtures of complex substances to start with, it can be inferred that the study of putrefactive changes is not a simple matter. On the whole, putrefaction can be characterized as a splitting up of complex organic molecules into more simple combinations. In some cases this will proceed far enough to result at last in the appearance of inorganic compounds like carbonic acid, sulphuretted hydrogen, ammonium salts, and free nitrogen. To get a fuller insight, however, into the chemistry of putrefaction, it would be necessary to follow the changes of every individual chemical substance of which the complex organic matter consists. Such a detailed study is at present foreign to our purpose. But to complete the definition, it must be added that the putrefactive changes are not due to any chemical or physical influences, other than the life-work of the microscopic beings present.

Confusion is apt to arise in the choice of the words putrefaction and fermentation. The latter term is not limited to the conversion of sugar into alcohol, though employed most commonly in that connection. Originally fermentation signifies a change started in a medium by the introduction of a minute quantity of some other substance, the change being often indicated by the formation of gas bubbles. The classical instance of a fermentation is of course the conversion of sugar into alcohol, and carbonic acid, the agent starting the process, the so-called ferment, being yeast. But we speak also of the acetic acid fermentation of alcohol, the lactic acid fermentation of sugars, and others. It will be shown later on that these fermentations are processes comparable to the putrefactive

changes. Hence no sharp line of distinction can be
drawn. Common usage perhaps prefers the word
fermentation when the resulting products are not
obnoxious to the nose, or are at least useful to man,
while closely allied changes, accompanied by a disagreeable smell, are termed rotting.

The invariable presence of bacteria in all putrefying
material suggests their close relation to that process,
but whether cause or result—can only be decided by
experiment, not by observation alone. The experimental proof, however, is so conclusive that it must be
accepted as an axiom, that no putrefaction can occur
without the presence of bacteria, and that bacteria are
the sole and only cause of such decomposition.

In order to demonstrate this truth, it has been
found most convenient to make use of clear solutions
of organic substances, for instance infusions of animal
or vegetable tissues. All that has been learned in
this manner applies equally to the decomposition of
the original solid substances, but it is not so convenient to demonstrate it. For in transparent solutions
bacteria can be detected more readily than on the
surface of solids. Moreover the occurrence, or absence,
of a turbidity in the previously clear fluid, is so suggestive of the presence of, or freedom from, bacteria,
that the microscope need not be appealed to in every
case. The first and most demonstrative result of such
observations has been that putrefaction is arrested by
any and all means, which arrest the development of
bacteria. For the present let us merely consider the
employment of heat for that purpose. Like all other
living beings bacteria are killed by a sufficient heat.
The boiling point of water is sufficient to kill all
bacteria (though, as we will learn later, the germs, or

seeds of some species resist even that temperature, and can thus cause errors on the part of observers). If hence an infusion of meat, or turnip, or cucumber, or beet, be boiled thoroughly and the vessel containing it be closed, so as to prevent the subsequent entrance of bacteria,· the solution will keep fresh indefinitely. No matter how long a time we allow to elapse, we will find no evidence of putrefaction on opening the vessel. Neither odor nor turbidity are observed, the microscope detects no bacteria and chemical analysis reveals no change. Another portion of the ·same infusion kept without being boiled, speedily decomposes. In some days at the latest, it will be found muddy, malodorous and teeming with bacterial life. The agent, therefore, which destroys the few bacteria pre-existing in the solution, has prevented that solution from spoiling. But the infusion thus preserved has not lost its aptitude for putrescence. For no matter how long it has been kept sweet, it will begin to undergo decomposition at once, as soon as we reintroduce bacteria into it. We can introduce a drop of another putrefying solution, or merely dip into it a needle previously in contact with rotten material. The transfer into it of the smallest practicable quantity of bacteria will start putrescence immediately. It is not even necessary to bring bacteria intentionally into the fluid; they are distributed throughout nature to such an extent that it is difficult to avoid introducing them unintentionally by contact with fingers, instruments or dust. On account of the analogy of this phenomenon to the communication of contagious diseases by contact with patients affected, we may also call the introduction of bacteria into a soil free of them *an infection*. But success in these simple and conclusive experiments has only been attained after patient research on the part of many observers.

The first condition for success in these experiments is the thorough purification of the glass vessels: i. e., the destruction of all bacteria adherent to the walls. If we resort to heat as the readiest agent .of destruction, we require an exposure of the whole vessel to a temperature of at least 150° C. for over an hour. On a small scale we can. succeed by heating a test tube momentarily to a higher degree with sufficient care in a large flame. The solution having been transferred into the prepared vessel, it is then boiled. Ordinarily a momentary boiling will suffice. But care must be taken that the fluid does not wet the sides of the glass and dry there in a thin layer. For any bacteria pre-existing in the fluid would now be subjected to the boiling heat in the dry state, in which state they are not killed with any certainty by that temperature. With sufficient attention to such details we can succeed in destroying all living organisms in the interior of the glass. This is technically called *sterilizing* the solution, and is the preparatory step in all such research. But such a solution will keep sterilized and sweet only under certain precautions; for instance, on sealing the flask. For experience has shown that all terrestrial objects have dried bacteria, or their germs. adhering to them, that bacteria constitute a part of all dust. Even avoiding all contact with objects impure in the sense of our experiments, we will find that no solution, however well sterilized, will keep long when exposed to the air. It is not difficult to show that the agent starting putrefaction in sterilized solutions is not gaseous, but consists of solid particles floating in the air. For as was first shown by Schroeder and Dusch (1854), air can be deprived of its power of starting decomposition by filtration through densely packed cotton. A sterilized solution can be kept forever unchanged by plugging the mouth of the bottle tightly with dry cotton. Pasteur, to whom we owe the most demonstrative experiments on this topic, has succeeded likewise in keeping solutions fresh by drawing out the neck of the flask into a long, thin and tortuous tube. The putrescible substances are thus fully exposed to the gases of the atmosphere, but any solid particles suspended in the air are caught in the meshes of the cotton, or deposited along the sides of Pasteur's narrow bent tubes. If we have once succeeded in destroying all germs in the flask and in the solution, neither bacteria nor any other living beings will ever be found in material thus preserved. Yet the most energetic decomposition, accompanied by the corresponding development of bacteria, will soon ensue upon removing the protecting plug of cotton, or snipping off the drawn-out neck of the flask. To put it in common parlance, wherever we sow bacteria in a proper soil we will reap a crop of bacteria. Prior to the researches just mentioned, it had been shown by Schwann * that the air could be rendered incapable of starting putrefaction by passing it through a highly heated tube. This indeed was the first proof that putrefaction can be started by a "something" in the air different from the gases. The solid particles which we now know to be the agents concerned, were simply burned in Schwann's experiments. Helmholtz, who has also worked on this subject, found, on the other hand, that pure oxygen obtained by electrolysis, could not provoke decomposition of sterilized fluids.

---

*Poggendorf's Annalen, 1837.

The floating matter in the air has been rendered visible by Tyndall* in an ingenious manner.

Who has not watched the motes dancing in the sunbeam, the track of which is revealed by their presence? The path of a ray of light is by itself not visible. We perceive the light only when it enters the eye. We see the bright spot on the wall where the sunbeam impinges, because it reflects some of the light into our eye. For the same reason a mote in the path of the light appears to us an illuminated speck. When the atmospheric dust consists of particles too fine to be seen separately, it causes the appearance of a cloudiness when struck by the beam of light. Tyndall made use of this principle and heightened its effect by causing a beam of strong light to pass through a chamber otherwise completely darkened. Under these circumstances the track of the ray appears luminous only if the air contains any floating particles. In many localities, at least in those where Tyndall experimented, the dust consists entirely of organic matter, and can be burned completely. A spirit lamp held under the luminous track of a lightbeam produces a gap in its continuity. The draught ascending from it contains no more solid particles, can reflect no more light and appears therefore intensely black, when compared with the light streak. If the air remains undisturbed in a case hermetically closed, all its dust will be found deposited on the sides of the box, after the lapse of a few days. By smearing the walls with glycerine Tyndall prevented the deposited particles from rising again. Through suitably arranged glass windows he could examine the path of a beam of sunlight or electric light traversing the

*Floating Matter of the Air, 1882.

box. This track became fainter and fainter, until at
last the absolute purity of the enclosed air was indicated by its perfect transparency. No light was inter-
cepted and scattered, for no floating particles existed
there, and the path of the ray could no longer be seen.
The same result could also be obtained in the course
of a few minutes by burning the dust of the enclosed
air by means of a wire heated with an electric current.

In the most elegant manner did Tyndall show that
this optically pure air, identical with the surrounding
air, but deprived of its dust, could not produce
decomposition. Test tubes had been let into the
bottom of such cases air-tight. They could be filled
through a movable pipette perforating a rubber
diaphragm in the top of the case, the entrance of the
pipette being protected by a packing of cotton. After
filling the glasses with various putrescible substances
and plugging the pipette, they were sterilized by five
minutes' boiling. Though exposed to the air in the
box these organic solutions kept sweet indefinitely,
while a second set of test tubes similarly filled and
similarly treated were teeming with life and most
offensive in .smell after a few days' exposure to the
impure air of the laboratory. Are not these various
experiments complete proof of the role of atmospheric
dust as a cause of putrefaction? Is there a link
wanting in the chain of evidence that the air cannot
by itself start decomposition, but that it contains
floating particles, living dust, which on reaching the
proper soil develop into the organisms whose life-
work reveals itself in putrefaction.

Yet this well-sustained doctrine of the origin of the
agents of putrefaction from germs suspended in the
air, has encountered much opposition at different times

in the past. It would be a waste of time to follow
in detail all the objections raised against it, to nar-
rate the numerous experiments apparently opposed to
it. For in every instance has later research by others
shown that such contradictory experiments were as
defective in their execution, as the conclusions drawn
from them were premature. No one now doubts the
relation of bacteria to putrefaction; no one claims that
decomposition ever occurs without lower organisms
living on dead material. But now and then a voice
is yet heard, maintaining that these organisms are
not necessarily introduced from without; that they can
arise without ancestors, can occur by new formation,
or *spontaneous generation*.

A historical survey shows us that the theory of
spontaneous generation was formerly applied to most
all lower animals, until their eggs were discovered by
advancing research. As the methods of observation
became more perfect, the field in which spontaneous
generation was supposed to prevail, was gradually
narrowed down, and now no one would dare to speak
of it except in connection with bacteria, the very
beings which tax the powers of the present micro-
scopes to the utmost. For a refutation of the older
champions of spontaneous generation I can refer you
to Cheyne's "Antiseptic Surgery," adding only that
former arguments have more recently been reproduced
and multiplied by Bastian.*

The strong point of these arguments is the appearance of bacteria in organic material *presumably
sterilized*, while apparently none have been introduced
from without. Hence it is claimed they must have
arisen from the dead organic substances, organic mole-

---

*Beginnings of Life, 1872.

cules have been revivified and have turned into
bacteria. Such a bold assertion, so opposed to all our
knowledge of life, requires unimpeachable proof,
which its promulgators are far from producing. The
chances of error in such research are numerous. In
the first place not one of the adherents of spontaneous
generation can or does claim to have purified his
flasks sufficiently in all instances. Usually the only
attempt at this indispensable precaution was the boiling of the contents after the glasses were filled.
This destroyed indeed all *developed bacteria pre-existing in the fluid*. But any *dried* germs adhering to
the walls of the flasks were not necessarily killed by
the heat of dry steam. We can heat desiccated germs
above 100° C. without depriving them of vitality.
Furthermore there is no guarantee that a brief boiling of the fluid will kill the germs suspended in the
air of the vessel. If a small amount of fluid is put
into a large flask there remains a large bulk of air
which it is not easy to purify. This seems to have
been the cause of the uncertainty of result obtained
by Wyman,* an impartial observer who did not deduce
unwarranted conclusions from his failure to maintain
his solutions free from germs and decomposition. All
experimenters who have been successful in proving the
stability of organic material when protected against
the germs in the air, agree, that their success became
constant only after learning the methods. Experience
taught them gradually what errors to avoid.

Bastian, the latest champion of spontaneous generation, or, as he calls it, "Archebiosis," claims that
the introduction of bits of cheese into the solutions
will invariably lead to the appearance of organisms in
spite of prolonged boiling. This fact as such has been

---

*Silliman's Journal, 1862 and 1867.

2

confirmed by Cohn,* who showed, however, that the organism appearing under these circumstances is invariably one and the same (viz: Bacillus subtilis), and that this bacterium will form *spores* or seeds which can withstand boiling for some time. The pre-existence of these spores in the cheese, where they have been actually demonstrated, is the clue to this alleged instance of spontaneous generation.

Tyndall has encountered similar instances of the resistance of spores to the heat of boiling water, but he has also shown how to destroy these spores.† For, when the fluid after boiling cools down to a proper temperature, *i. e.* about 30° to 40° C., these spores will germinate. In the *developed* state the resulting bacteria are easily killed by heat, even less than that of boiling water. Hence a brief boiling *repeated* at intervals of several hours, never fails to ·sterilize a solution. And thus all arguments to the effect that bacteria can appear in the interior of closed flasks after boiling can be overthrown by Tyndall's methods of repeated boiling.

It has been urged that the existence of spontaneous generation cannot be disproven by the permanent sterility of boiled fluids, for we do not know in what way heat may interfere with the new formation of living beings, an argument ˙which must be respected until disproven by experiment. Observations, however, on the part of Van der Broeck, of Roberts and others have shown, that substances as putrescible as grape juice, and the tissues of various vegetables, will not putrefy at all if received in glass tubes previously heated. In these experiments these substances themselves were neither heated nor in any other way acted

---

*Beitraege z. Biologie d. Pflanzen, Bd. I., Heft 3, p. 188.

†Floating Matter, etc., p. 210.

upon, but simply removed and kept with precautions preventing the access of germs. For no bacteria can be found in the interior of living plants and animals. It will be shown later on that also the animal fluids, blood and urine, so readily alterable when exposed to the air, can be preserved fresh indefinitely, if only protected against sources of external infection. Hence there remains really no proof whatever, that spontaneous generation can ever occur under any circumstances with which we are acquainted.

It is necessary to have some system under which to classify the various forms of bacteria met with. Different systems have been proposed, of which the best one is that of Cohn.* It is based only on the forms of these beings, and according to their shape it recognizes them as,

　I. SPHÆROBACTERIA (round granules).

　II. MICROBACTERIA (short rods).

　III. DESMOBACTERIA (straight filaments).

　IV. SPIROBACTERIA (spiral filaments).

Each of these groups is then further subdivided into separate species. Usage, however, amongst the most reliable authors has further simplified this classification, so that now the word bacteria is used commonly in a generic sense, while three subdivisions are recognized, termed, according to the form, (1) *Micrococcus*, (2) *Bacillus* and (3) *Spirillum*.

Micrococci, or, simply cocci, identical with Cohn's Sphærobacteria, are granules either round or elliptical, of about one half to two micromillimeters in diameter, or even smaller. According to a rather cumbersome nomenclature introduced by Billroth,† we speak of diplo-coccus when two granules adhere together in

---

*Beitraege zur Biologie der Pflanzen, Bd. I., Zweites Heft, p. 146.

†Untersuchungen ueber d. Vegetations-formen von Coccobacteria septica, 1874.

dumb-bell form, and of streptococcus when a series
of them are joined, forming a chain. Quite commonly micrococci collect in groups, sometimes pretty
large, held together by a matrix of mucous-like or
gelatinous consistency. This is called the Zoogloea
form (Billroth's Gliacoccus).

Bacilli are, as the name indicates, rods. The distinction between the short rods constituting Cohn's
Microbacteria and the longer threads—really chains
of rods—which he terms Desmobacteria, has not
been maintained by usage, because impracticable.
Bacilli have a length of from one to six micromillimeters, or even beyond. Their diameter may be
as much as one, or even two micromillimeters, but is
sometimes so small as to be unmeasurable. The
French use the word vibrio for bacillus, though this
term is often employed indiscriminately. Bacilli
may take the zoogloea form but are oftener found
in dense "swarms" without the gelatinous basis.
Some varieties do not segment or separate, or separate only imperfectly in segments, as they grow,
and thus form thread-like chains. When the segmentation of the chains is distinct they are sometimes termed Leptothrix.

Spirilla is the common term for the Spirobacteria of
Cohn, though he distinguishes between spirochæte, a
screw-shaped thread with flexible and narrow coil,
and the spirillum, a more rigid and wider screw.
Spirilla represent threads twisted in the form of a
screw, with from one to four or five turns; their
length may be four to fifteen micromillimeters, with
a diameter of the convolutions from two to three
micromillimeters. Some giant forms, however, are
met with of nearly three times the largest of these
dimensions. Spirilla occur only singly, or in densely

matted clusters. It seems very questionable to me
whether spirilla really belong to the bacteria. For, as
regards their mode of reproduction nothing certain is
known, while both in their shape, as well as in their
behavior to staining agents they differ radically from
other bacteria. Since we will have but little occasion to refer again to the order of spirilla, except
with reference to two kinds found only in the human
body, it may be well to state here, that different
representatives of this family are encountered in
many stagnant waters. It is not known that they
exert any action upon the soil in which they vegetate comparable to putrefaction or fermentation.

LECTURE II.

The Examination of Bacteria.—Staining Methods.—Illumination with
Abbe's Condensor.—Structure of Bacteria.—The Flagellum.—Bacterial Movements.—Reproduction.—Spores and their Vitality and
Power of Resistance.—Composition of Bacteria.—Bacterial Food.
Oxygen.—"Fermentation is Life without Free Oxygen."—Aerobes
and Anærobes.—The Influence of Temperature upon Bacteria and
their Spores.—Desiccation.—Germs in the Air.

The examination of living bacteria is often unsatisfactory, on account of their minuteness and transparency.
In many cases also their motion interferes with close
observation. Save a few striking forms it is scarcely
possible to identify different bacteria examined fresh.
It was hence no slight merit on the part of Koch to
perfect a method facilitating bacterial examinations.
Instead of viewing them suspended in fluids, Koch
spreads the fluid containing them in the thinnest layer
possible on an ordinary cover glass, and dries it.*
The bacteria are not distorted and do not shrink by
drying, but retain their natural appearance, and indeed
appear more striking in air than in fluids of about
the same index of refraction as the bacterial body
itself. In order to prevent this dried spot from redis-
solving on the application of staining agents it must

---

*Beitraege zur Biologie der Pflanzen, Bd. II., Heft III., p. 399.

be rendered insoluble by the action of absolute alcohol. Still more convenient, as Koch has since shown, is the hardening influence of heat by drawing the specimen a few times through a gas or spirit flame. The best staining of bacteria can be accomplished with aniline colors, in moderately concentrated aqueous solution, for instance, methyl violet (blue ink), methyl green, magenta, and many others. Aniline brown in glycerine solution (half glycerine, half water) is also useful, especially in the case of bacteria in albuminous fluids, or for photographic purposes. A drop of the aniline solution is placed upon the dried spot on the cover glass and left there some minutes. The time of exposure varies with the concentration of the dye, and the kind of bacteria. The solution is now washed off with a jet of water and the glass is dried, if desirable with the aid of gentle heat. The specimen can be examined in water, or mounted permanently in Canada balsam. In successful mountings the bacteria alone should be stained. In order to perceive well the color of such minute objects, no diaphragm with narrow aperture can be used beneath the stage of the microscope; on the contrary, the more diffuse the illumination, the more striking does the color appear.

In the midst of animal tissues the detection of bacteria is a more difficult matter than in fluids. Formerly sections of tissues were treated with acetic acid, or solution of potassic hydrate, whereby any colonies of bacteria were indeed rendered more apparent, on account of the greater transparency of the other tissues. But in the case of single bacteria scattered throughout the tissue, this method is of little use. The staining of bacteria, especially with aniline colors, as introduced by Weigert, was therefore quite an improvement. Certain manipulations, however,

are necessary to produce good staining. Tissues must
be hardened in alcohol preparatory to cutting into thin
sections. The sections are then put into strong watery
solutions of aniline colors, methyl-violet, magenta,
brown, or others. In his most recent publication*
Weigert recommends especially gentian-violet in one
per cent. solution as the most reliable staining agent.
Methyl-blue has also been lauded highly by Ehrlich.
Experience must show how long the individual section
is to remain in the dye—some minutes, or many hours.
After sufficient staining, the sections are washed in
water and decolorized in dilute acetic acid, or as
Weigert now prefers it in neutral absolute alcohol,
which extracts the color out of all parts but the
nuclei and the micro-organisms present. They are then
mounted in the usual manner in Canada balsam. In
such specimens only bacteria and cell nuclei are
stained, and therefore attract the eye. But in the
case of very small bacteria, when scattered throughout
the tissue, the amount of color is too slight to be
recognized, except with a special mode of illumination
introduced by Koch.†

It is only by the aid of this method that the systematic detection of bacteria in animal tissues is possible.
The principle of this method is the following: The
microscopic image of uncolored objects depends for
its formation upon differences in the refractive indices
of the component parts of the object. If the different fibres and cells of a colorless section had the same
common index of refraction—that is, produced the same
deviation throughout of the rays of light passing

---

*Virchow's Archiv, Bd. 84, p. 275.

†Investigations into the Etiology of Traumatic Infective Diseases.
Translated by W. Watson Cheyne. Sydenham Society: 1880. p. 24.
(The German original appeared in 1878.)

through them, no structure could be seen.   It is only
because the different rays *are* refracted differently by
the different parts of the object, that an image is
formed of light and shadow.   This image is most
pronounced when the rays of light which illuminate
the object from below are parallel, while the more
diffuse the illumination the more effaced is the distinction between light and shadow in the image.   But
all this does not apply to the image of colored objects.
In this case the brighter the light the more striking
is the color.   The image of stained microscopic objects
is thus made up of the structure-image and the color-
image.   If the former is well developed by illumination through only a narrow diaphragm beneath the
microscopic stage it can hide feebler details in the
color-image, for instance, isolated bacteria moderately
stained.   Hence, in order to bring out best the pure
color-image, the structure-image should be effaced by
the most diffuse illumination possible.   This can be
best accomplished by means of an Abbe's condensor,
a combination of lenses below the stage, having a
short focal range and wide aperture.   The object is
thus flooded with light to such an extent that the
structure and contours almost disappear, while any
stained particles, no matter how small, stand forth
prominently.

It is only since the introduction of Koch's methods
of examination, that we can identify individual bacteria
with certainty.   Prior to this, the most confusing
errors had been committed in the description of
bacteria.   Since the distinction between different
species depends often upon minute differences in the
dimensions, and upon peculiarities in the form, which
seem so insignificant as to scarcely attract the eye,
it is evident that the most conscientious drawings

of such minute objects are unreliable for identification. It is only the photograph which can be accepted as unimpeachable evidence in a comparison of the forms observed by different authors. Again we are under the greatest obligations to Dr. Koch for perfections in the photographic reproduction of bacteria.

The examination of bacteria, either living or stained, reveals no further structure. No cell wall can be recognized with certainty. No nucleus is ever seen. The body appears to be homogenous protoplasm. In some instances, however, a whip-like cord, the *flagellum*, is found as a prolongation of the body of certain rod-shaped bacteria at either end. In the larger spirilla this structure is distinct enough to be recognized tolerably easily, especially when it is not in too violent motion. For the flagellum is the organ of motion comparable to the cilia of the lower animals. The flagella of bacilli, however, are so delicate as to be scarcely recognizable, though with good lenses and very oblique illumination they have been seen in even the smaller forms (Bacterium termo) by Dollinger and Drysdale.* Koch has shown that the flagellum becomes more distinct in the dried specimen. He obtained the best result, however, by staining the specimen on the cover glass with concentrated aqueous extract of logwood. It is rendered more striking by subsequent treatment with chromic acid solution. Aniline colors will not stain the flagellum. No flagella have ever been seen in any specimen of micrococcus.

Many forms of bacteria are in a state of continual motion during life which interferes, of course, with close observation. It is necessary to distinguish between purely passive movements and the locomotion

---

*Monthly Microscopical Journal, Sept. 1875

due to the vital contractions of the bacterial body.
The passive motion is identical in nature with the
molecular or Brownian movements observable in all
sufficiently small particles suspended in a limpid fluid.
When an alcoholic solution of shellac is precipitated
by the addition of water, the minutely divided particles of shellac are seen under the microscope to be in a
state of constant trembling and dancing movement,
being carried hither and thither by faint currents in
the fluid in which they are suspended. The molecular
agitation is intensified by radiant heat. This Brownian
movement explains why very fine precipitates settle
with such slowness, especially when not protected
against light and heat. This passive movement can
involve dead bacteria as well as living ones. It is
hence not stopped by the action of poisons. The
Brownian movement is observed in all micrococci not
united in chains or groups. Indeed, in most cases
micrococci possess only this passive movement, though
in inaccurate descriptions they have often been spoken
of as actively moving. Yet some varieties, for instance
the micrococcus found by Ogston in pus, present a
motion, which must be recognized as of the active
order. The Brownian movement involves also the
smaller forms of rod-shaped bacteria. In very viscid
fluids these movements are checked.

Quite different from this passive agitation is the
active locomotion by which bacilli and spirilla and
some forms of micrococci shoot to and fro in the field.
With eel-like flexions these organisms propel themselves, now slowly, then rapidly, and suddenly change
direction, often with a precision comparable to the
voluntary motion of animals. At the same time rotation around the axis of the body is often seen, especially when this axis forms an acute angle with the

axis of the microscope. These movements are accomplished mainly by aid of the flagella, though the sinuous twisting of the body must also play some part. The active movements are of course stopped by any poison or agent killing the bacteria. Yet arrest of this motion is not necessarily indicative of death, for the bacteria may be benumbed and still recover, for instance, by extreme cold or heat. Moreover many forms of bacilli *never* show these movements, while other species possess motion only during a part of their life-time.

The only absolute criterion of the life of bacteria is their power of multiplication. Under proper conditions of nourishment and temperature each granule or rod elongates and then divides into two. When the young organisms thus formed remain attached to each other partially or wholly, chains and threads are produced. If the division occurs in more than one direction groups are formed. The substance constituting the basis of zoogloea masses is probably derived by transformation of the outer part of the bacterial body. The multiplication by *fission* continues until the soil is exhausted, or until the waste products of the bacterial tissue-change accumulate to a poisonous extent. The terrific rate of reproduction of these micro-organisms can be better appreciated by quoting some figures from Cohn. Observation has shown that a bacterial generation can arise in the course of about one, hour. At this rate a single bacterium would produce two in one hour; these by doubling would increase to four in the second hour, and so on—until after the lapse of three days the scarcely conceivable figure of 4772 billions would be attained. A single bacterium termo is a rod about one micromillimeter thick, and twice as long. Assum-

ing the specific gravity of the bacterial body to be
equal to that of water it would require 636000 millions of bacteria for the weight of one milligram.
But a single bacterium could raise a progeny within
twenty-four hours equalling in weight $\frac{1}{80}$ milligram,
while the bacterial family with a pedigree reaching
back three days, would balance the scales at $7\frac{1}{2}$
million kilograms (7500 tons). In reality this scarcely
credible rate of reproduction is not maintained long
from want of nourishment. Yet a growth not far
behind these marvellous figures can be observed when
bacteria invade a solid soil—for instance, a cooked
potato. The merest speck with which the soil is
infected, will grow at the proper temperature at such
a rate, that within a day the whole potato is transformed into a bacterial mass.

Fission is not the only mode of reproduction of
bacteria. Propagation by spores can be observed in
all the larger forms of bacilli, but has not yet been
seen in some of the smaller species of rods, nor in
micrococci. The formation of spores is a criterion by
which we can assign bacteria to the vegetable kingdom, for in animals we never observe the appearance
of germs coincident with the death of the parent,
which mode of reproduction is quite common amongst
plants. Sporification always alternates with fission.
As far as observation goes, young bacilli invariably
grow and multiply by division for some time before
they produce spores. Continued vegetation without
change of soil is usually terminated by the formation
of spores, and these spores will not as a rule germinate in the unchanged soil where they were produced.
The conditions, however, governing sporification are
not fully understood. The process has been best
studied in the *bacillus anthracis* (the parasite of

splenic fever), and in a similar organism, encountered on the surface of hay, the *bacillus subtilis*. At a certain stage in the life of these bacilli there appear faint granules in the interior of the rods which change gradually into brilliant oval spots nearly as wide as the original rod. Of these there may be from one to five in a row in each bacillus. During this time the bacterial body becomes fainter and disintegrates, until finally the spores separate, each being surrounded by a fine halo, probably of protoplasm. In some instances the spores are held together by this mass, like a string of beads. In other species of bacilli the spores are not always so highly refractive and brilliant as in the instances described. They may also appear at the ends of the rod instead of in its interior, but these forms have not been so well studied. Ordinarily spores are immovable. But I have seen some spores, probably of the bacillus, which causes buytric acid fermentation, shoot to and fro in a manner which could only have been produced by a powerful flagellum, though I could not recognize the latter. On account of the similarity in form and size, individual spores cannot be distinguished with certainty from single micrococci. But unlike micrococci they are not stained, as a rule, by aniline colors.

Spores are characterized by a much greater resistance to damaging influences than the adult bacteria. They can withstand higher temperatures, and are killed only by very few poisons. As long as the spores do not germinate they are practically immortal as far as time is concerned, which is true also of many other vegetable seeds. The transformation of the vulnerable bacteria into the almost indestructible permanent form of spores explains the persistence of the species under unfavorable circumstances. When placed into the proper soil and kept at favorable temperature the spores germinate within a few hours. The oval granule elongates in one direction, loses its brilliancy, and is thus converted into a young bacillus which keeps on growing and dividing. As soon as the germination is complete, the remarkable resisting power of the spore is lost. If thus the spores are difficult to kill by continuous boiling, heating at intervals according to the method of Tyndall will effectually sterilize any soil by giving the spores time to germinate and attacking the bacteria in their least resisting form.

Like all living beings bacteria can grow only at the expense of the food which they consume. In any soil in which they do not find sufficient nourishment they cease to grow. What substances they require can be inferred from the composition of their bodies. The only analysis published of bacterial protoplasm is by Nencki and Schaffer.* The bacteria (evidently the common forms of putrefaction) growing in gelatine solution were isolated by boiling with 2 to 3 per cent. of hydrochloric acid, after which procedure they could be filtered off. The bacterial mass contained 85 per cent. of water. Of the solids 85 per cent. were albuminoids; the fats amounted to 6 to 7 per cent., and the ashes to 3 or 4 per cent. About two per cent. of the solids was not definitely recognized, probably cellulose. The albumen of bacteria, which the authors propose to call myko-protin, differs slightly in its properties from animal and vegetable albuminoids. As a matter of special interest Nencki points out that it contains less nitrogen than other albuminoid substances, only 13.65 per cent. (instead of 15 to 16 per

---

*Journal f. pract. Chemie. Vol. 20, 1879, p. 443.

cent). In bacterial colonies in the form of zoogloea
masses the authors found no chemical differences.
They hence consider the zoogloea the transformed
bacterial bodies and not a separate substance.

A solution intended for the growth of bacteria must
contain the necessary salts, viz.: phosphates and
sulphates of potassium and magnesium (perhaps also
calcium). They can be either chemically free or
combined with some of the organic principles. The
albumen need not pre-exist as such in the solution.
Like all plants bacteria (at least some species of
them) can build up their albumen from simpler nitrogenous compounds. Indeed, this faculty of forming
albumen synthetically is one of the criteria by means
of which bacteria are assigned to the vegetable kingdom. The simplest chemical substances from which
bacteria can elaborate their nitrogenous principles are
the salts of ammonia with vegetable acids. Although
fats and hydrocarbons form part of the bacterial
protoplasm, they need not be furnished as such; they
can be formed at the expense of the albumen or its
elements. Hence bacteria can thrive actively in fluids
of very simple composition, which contain only a
compound of ammonia with a vegetable acid, besides
the necessary salts. Such a fluid is usually termed a
cultivating solution. The first one devised by Pasteur,
which yet bears his name, consists of 10 parts of
crystallized sugar, and 1 part of tartrate of ammonium,
and the ashes of 1 part of yeast (about 0.075 parts
per weight) in 100 parts of distilled water. The
sugar was added because the mixture was intended
originally for the nutrition of yeast, but it is not
necessary for the growth of bacteria. Cohn's solution,
also much used, has the following formula: Distilled
water, 20.; Tartrate of Ammonium, 0.2; Phosphate of

Potassium, 0.1; Sulphate of Magnesium, 0.1; Basic Phosphate of Calcium, 0.01.

While these proportions need not be accurately maintained, experience has shown, that they are the most favorable on the whole. But it must not be supposed that such mineral solutions, since they permit the growth of bacteria, are necessarily the best soil for them. Although bacteria can build up their organic principles from simpler molecules, they thrive much better, when a more elaborate food is offered them. An infusion of almost any vegetable or animal tissue is by far a better soil for them than these mineral solutions. This is quite apparent from the fact that such infusions become turbid speedily when exposed to the air, while Pasteur's or Cohn's solutions are not readily infected by the germs of atmospheric dust. It is only when bacteria already developed are sown in these solutions, that they will multiply. Probably the acid reaction of these mineral solutions is by itself unfavorable to bacteria, which thrive best in alkaline soil. But even this hindrance removed, such mineral solutions cannot nourish those species of bacteria accustomed to living in the animal body. Adapted as these forms are to a parasitic mode of life, they are not able to build their organic principles by synthesis. Many of them will not grow in any soil which does not closely resemble in composition the animal juices. Many authors have committed the most confusing errors by attempting to cultivate disease germs in mineral solutions, in which they could find no nourishment. Under these circumstances the occurrence of a turbidity could have been due only to the accidental introduction of other germs.

The relation of bacteria to oxygen is as yet involved in much uncertainty. Some of the forms

3

occurring in the common putrefactive processes consume oxygen and exhale carbonic acid like other
living beings. This fact can be demonstrated by
gasometric analysis in any closed vessel in which they
vegetate. The influence of oxygen on the life of such
bacteria, as manifested in their movements, has been
studied experimentally by Grossmann and Mayerhausen.*
A cover-glass, on the lower side of which there was a
drop of fluid containing bacteria, was used as the cover
of a microscopic gas chamber. Bacteria were thus
observed while different gases were passed through
the chamber. The movements were most energetic
when the bacteria were exposed to pure oxygen, and
ceased after a while, whenever this agent was replaced
by any other gas. Lately the influence of oxygen
upon bacterial movement has even been suggested by
Engelmann as the most delicate test for free oxygen.
On placing on the same slide putrefactive bacteria
together with vegetable cells containing chlorophyll,
and varying the intensity of the illumination, the
bacteria indicated by their active motion, whenever the
green plant cells liberated oxygen under the influence
of light.

While the want of active movement during the
absence of oxygen does not necessarily signify the
death of the bacteria, it has been shown that the
prolonged deprivation of oxygen does kill certain
bacteria as well as higher species of living beings.
In the case of the organism concerned in the fermentation of urine, as well as the bacterial parasite of
splenic fever, reproduction ceases after deprivation of
oxygen.

While thus some bacteria require oxygen like other

forms of life, there are other species differing entirely
in this respect. Pasteur was the first to show that
under some circumstances life can continue without
free oxygen. He demonstrated this in the case of the
yeast plant, which is commonly classed amongst the
fungi. This being can live with, or without, free
oxygen. It grows most energetically when exposed to
oxygen, though its development does not cease completely when deprived of it. Its chemical activity,
however, as manifested by the conversion of the
sugary soil in which it lives into alcohol, is most
marked in the absence of oxygen. This statement
once disputed by Brefeld and by Traube, has subsequently been confirmed by them upon further research.
Pasteur, indeed, denies even that the yeast cell causes
fermentation at all, when it can get free oxygen,
claiming that in a fermenting solution exposed to the
air, the oxygen is consumed in the lower strata before
the fermentation begins. He formulates his views in
the famous statement that "fermentation is life without free oxygen." He explains in fact the fermentative action of the yeast cell by its avidity for oxygen.
For when the latter element is not present in the free
state, the yeast cell procures the oxygen it needs at
the expense of the substances which it can split up.
Although it would seem that no oxygen could be
seized by the yeast when it splits up sugar into
alcohol and carbonic acid, still this is not strictly true.
For Pasteur showed that really a part of the sugar is
transformed into other products, viz: glycerine, succinic
acid, etc., and thereby yields oxygen to the yeast.
Pasteur proved, furthermore, that also some other
beings, for instance the mould-fungi known as Mucor,
can ferment sugar when deprived of oxygen, but have
not that property when exposed to air. However, it

would be 'foreign to our topic to discuss all of
Pasteur's ingenious observations on yeast, and their
conclusiveness. For further details I must refer you
to his instructive "Studies on Fermentation."*

On extending his observations to bacteria, Pasteur
found that some of these as well can exist without
free oxygen. He claimed this originally for the
bacillus concerned in butyric acid fermentation, but
subsequently showed it to be true of certain other
species. Not only are the fermentative changes due
to these organisms impossible in the presence of oxygen,
but the very movements of such bacteria are checked
by that gas, and their development hindered.

Pasteur hence recognizes amongst bacteria two
classes, the *Aerobes* and the *Anaerobes.* The former
require free oxygen, the latter cannot live in its pressure. According to the views of Pasteur only
anaerobic bacteria, or at least such forms as can
temporarily exist without free oxygen, produce the
changes of putrefaction and fermentation. The facts,
however, which Pasteur adduces are neither numerous
enough nor sufficiently convincing to prove the theory
that fermentation is always life without free oxygen.
The principal fact, however, upon which Pasteur bases
his theory, viz: that at least certain bacteria can live,
multiply, and produce fermentative changes, without
the presence of free oxygen, has been fully substan-
tiated by others. Huefner† showed that putrefaction
can occur in a vacuum by inclosing putrescible substances in a flask, the narrow neck of which was bent
horizontally and closed hermetically after all air had
been expelled by boiling the fluid. A drop of
bacterial fluid had previously been placed in a hollow

*English Translation by Faulkner and Robb, 1879.
†Journal f. pract. Chemie. Vol. 13, (1876) p. 475.

·depression in the bent neck of the flask, so that the organisms could not be killed by the steam. On inverting the flask the bacteria were brought into the boiled contents. On opening the flask after some ·days, the contents were rotten and teeming with bacteria. But no description is given of their form. Subsequently Jeanneret and Nencki* repeated similar experiments with the same result. The putrefaction proceeded about six times as slowly as it did in the presence of oxygen, but the chemical products of the decomposition of gelatine or albumen were the same, whether oxygen was present or not. The validity of these observations was contested by Gunning† on the ground that the last traces of oxygen cannot be removed from a fluid by either boiling or the action of an air pump. For even under these circumstances a delicate reaction for oxygen can still be obtained, by means of the bluing of a mixture of ferrous sulphate with yellow prussiate of potassium in solution, with the addition of a drop of a solution of hypo-sulphite of sodium. That such a minute trace of oxygen must be taken into consideration with refer-ence to bacterial tissue change, he tries to render evident by the following figures. If we assume the weight of a single large bacterium to be $\frac{1}{2500000000}$ milligram, and if from analogy with higher beings we admit that bacteria consume about 1 per cent. of their weight of oxygen in 24 hours, one million bacteria would require at the most $\frac{1}{25000}$ milligram, i. e., approximately $\frac{1}{30000}$ cubic centimeters of oxygen. But Gunning overlooks the enormous num-bers of bacteria existing in putrid solutions. Any one familiar with the microscopic appearance of blood,

---

*Journal f. pract. Chemie. Vol. 15, p. 353.
†Journal f. pract. Chemie. Vol. 16, p. 314, and Vol. 17, p. 266.

must admit that in any rotting solution bacteria are many times more numerous than are the red corpuscles in the blood. Since of the latter there are five millions in every cubic millimeter of blood, thirty millions bacteria per cubic millimeter of a putrid fluid is certainly a low estimate. At this rate, and on the basis of Gunning's figures, the putrid solution would consume its equal bulk of oxygen in twenty-four hours.

The possibility of putrefaction without free oxygen has indeed been shown by Nencki* in later and more elaborate experiments in which the absence of oxygen was guaranteed by the presence of an alkaline solution of pyrogallic acid in a separate portion of the set of bent tubes employed. This fluid would have absorbed any traces of oxygen, and indicated this occurrence by turning brown. The putrefaction was brought to a stand-still after a time if the volatile products of decomposition were prevented from escaping. But when these substances were allowed to escape through a tube dipped into a solution of pyrogallic acid in order to prevent the entrance of oxygen, the process continued without air. Under these circumstances, however, other forms of bacteria were found than in a soil exposed to the atmosphere. Nencki saw principally a form of micrococcus, and, to less extent, long bacilli. This agrees with the observation that in ordinary rotting fluids the shorter rods abound on the surface where they can procure oxygen, while in the deeper strata not reached by that gas, micrococci vegetate mainly.

The behavior of bacteria towards oxygen varies also with reference to its allotropic form, viz: ozone. While this gas kills certain bacteria of putrefaction at once, as was shown by their disintegration in the

---

*Journal f. pract. Chemie. Vol. 19, p. 337.

experiments of Grossmann and Mayerhausen, it does not seem to harm the bacilli of splenic fever blood. Of further observations with this gas I can find no account. Common oxygen, however, when compressed to a tension of five atmospheres is fatal to all living beings, as Paul Bert has shown in his fascinating experiments on compressed air. Bacteria are not exceptions to this universal reaction; they are killed at once by this agent in its compressed condition. But the spores of bacteria can resist this poisonous influence; of all living matter they are the most difficult to destroy. Hence, Bert could not realize the hope of distinguishing between the processes due to bacterial life, and the changes produced by chemical ferments, by means of oxygen at a high pressure. For although the soluble ferments are not hindered in their action by compressed oxygen, the spores will likewise resist, and can afterwards germinate under proper conditions.

When bacteria are sown in proper soil, their rate of development and their chemical energy depend upon the temperature. At low temperatures bacteria are benumbed; as soon as warmth is applied they re-awake, and their vital energy is then commensurate to the temperature up to a certain limit, beyond which they are again benumbed and ultimately killed. Extreme cold does not seem able to destroy all bacteria, for in the experiments of Frisch, exposure to 110° C. below zero did not kill the bacillus of splenic fever blood. According to Eidam* the bacteria of putrefaction (B. termo) begin their movements and multiplication at 5½° C. The vital energy then proceeds proportionate to the temperature up to 35° C.; beyond this it again flags and at 40° C. the

---

*Cohn's Beitraege z. Biologie d. Pflanzen, Bd. I, Heft III, p. 208.

condition of heat torpor ensues. These limits of
temperature are not the same for all bacteria. The
bacilli found on the surface of hay can yet grow
between 47° and 50° C. according to Cohn, but
their development is arrested above this point. In
fact the larger spore-producing bacilli seem more
resistant than the smaller organisms. The formation
of spores cannot take place below 15° to 18° C.
(Koch), and is checked again by a temperature
probably variable with the different species. Pasteur
claims that 43° C. prevents sporification in the
case of the bacilli of splenic fever. This limit probably varies with the nature of the medium in which
they grow, since Koch has seen spores form at this
temperature. The hay-bacillus ceased to produce
spores only at 50° C. when cultivated in an infusion of hay by Cohn*.

No adult bacteria have as yet been found to
survive after long exposure to 60° C. when in the
moist state. Even a lower thermal limit than this has
been found to destroy some bacteria. Eidam killed
bacterium termo by 14 hours' exposure to 45° C.,
or by the action of 50° C. during three hours,
while Chauveau destroyed the life of the more
resistant splenic fever bacillus by an exposure to
50° C. for only 20 minutes. Many contradictory
results, however, have been recorded on account of
inaccuracy of the methods. The submersion of a test
tube filled with the bacterial cultivating fluid in an
open water bath heated to the desired degree does
not guarantee that the bacteria are really exposed to
the temperature of the water bath. Under such
circumstances the poor conductivity of the glass tube
and of the water, the evaporation of fluid from the

*Beitraege z. Biologie d. Pflanzen, Bd. II., Heft II, p. 249.

surface of the bacterial liquid, and the cooling influence of currents of air above the surface, these all prevent the bacterial soil from reaching the temperature of the surrounding bath, at least for an uncertain length of time. The only reliable method is the one followed by Chauveau, viz: to inclose a relatively small quantity of the bacterial fluid in a *thin-walled closed* pipette, and to suspend this in the interior of the water bath. This observer did thus really find a low temperature to suffice for the destruction of the micro-organisms, because they were *actually* heated to this point (50° C.).

The spores of bacteria can undoubtedly resist a much higher degree of temperature than suffices for the destruction of the developed forms. All observers agree that the boiling point of water is the lowest limit to be relied upon for their annihilation. Thus Fitz* found that the spores of a bacillus producing the butyric fermentation of glycerine were killed with certainty by 3 to 20 minutes' boiling, while it required 2 to 6 hours to destroy them at 95° C. and 7 to 11 hours at 80° C. According to the last researches by Koch† the spores of the splenic fever parasite, as well as of the different bacilli found in the surface soil of the earth, are infallibly killed by 100° C. But while the former yield after two minutes' boiling, the earth spores resist up to 10 to 15 minutes. Convinced by the uniformity of his own results Koch ventures to state, that probably all spores die at 100° C., provided only that they are really exposed to that temperature. For in the numerous contradictory observations by other authors a guarantee was not always given, that

---

*Berichte d. deutschen chemischen Gesellschaft, Vol. 15, p. 867, 1882.

†Mittheilungen a. d. Kaiserl. Gesundheitsamte. 1881. p. 322.

the spores were really heated to the point stated. In the case of test tubes immersed in a water bath — the method most commonly used—the reasons above stated why the bacteria did not reach the temperature of the water bath hold good, as Koch has shown by thermometric measurement. He demonstrated likewise that even inside of closed boilers, filled flasks exposed to the contained steam do not reach the temperature of the compressed steam, until after the lapse of a long time proportionate to the size of the flask. Moreover, if the fluid containing spores spurts, some of the spores may dry on the side of the vessel above the level of the fluid, and *dry* spores are not killed by 100° C. Hence Koch regards with suspicion all former statements that spores can resist prolonged boiling. Yet Tyndall* states that he has boiled hay infusions for hours (in one case even 8 hours) without being able to sterilize them, apparently with the utmost accuracy of method. It is also claimed by Pasteur that, in alkaline fluids, spores are not killed with certainty by boiling at the atmospheric pressure. Milk, however, which in the earlier experiments of Schroeder could not be sterilized at 100° C., Pasteur succeeded in keeping pure by prolonged boiling. At any rate, wet spores can be inevitably killed by a few minutes' exposure to 110° C. (under pressure).

In the dried state bacteria are less readily destroyed by heat. The experience of most observers has shown this to be a fact, but I can find no definite statements as regards the least temperature requisite to kill the developed forms. In the experiments of Koch all adult bacteria were destroyed by an hour's sojourn in a hot-air chamber in which the temperature rose at last to about 120° C. Spores, however, were not

---

*Floating Matter, etc., p. 199.

injured under these circumstances. Their resistance was only overcome by three hours' exposure to 140° C.

Drying by itself does not immediately destroy the life of bacteria. Spores in this condition are practically imperishable, but in the case of the developed forms the possibility of a return to the living condition when moistened again, does not seem to persist forever. From statements by various authors it is to be inferred that the length of time during which this dormant vitality of the dried bacteria can last varies in different species. According to the precise statements of Koch the bacillus of splenic fever lost its vitality inside of 12 to 30 hours when well dried in thin layers, but in thicker masses, not completely desiccated, it survived during some weeks.

Further studies of the influence of desiccation upon the life of bacteria are required, in order to explain in what form germs exist in the air.

Bodies of such minute size as bacteria have such an immense surface compared with their bulk, that they must speedily dry and shrivel, when floating in an air not saturated with aqueous vapor. How long the developed forms can survive under these circumstances we do not know, though the spores are not injured whatsoever, judging from all experiments to the point. Microscopic examination of the air is rather unsatisfactory. The atmospheric dust does, of course, settle upon a slide and can be collected in a drop of glycerine, or other adhesive fluid, and then examined, but numerous observations made thus by different authors have taught very little. The shrivelled bacteria cannot be easily recognized and certainly not identified; moreover, it can not be decided by the microscope, whether the dried specimen is dead or yet capable of development. A better method to get an insight into the nature of

the atmospheric dust is to expose to it a nutritive soil
in which the bacteria deposited by the air can develop.
Of course, due care must be taken to previously sterilize thoroughly this soil, and the vessels in which it
is contained. The speediness with which bacteria
appear, and the forms observed, indicate their distribution in the air, but not the condition in which they
existed there. In his now classical observations, Pasteur* learned thus, that the tops of uninhabited
mountains were · surrounded by an atmosphere containing but few germs. Similar has also been the
experience of Tyndall. In undisturbed vaults Pasteur
found also a scantiness of aerial germs, the quietude
and want of ventilation favoring the subsidence of all
suspended matter. The existence of much dust in the
air does not necessarily indicate a corresponding abundance of germs, for on open roads the dust may be
largely mineral or soot. · But in laboratories where
investigations on germs have long been carried on, the
air becomes infected finally to an extent compromising
further research. After Tyndall had handled hay in
his laboratory for some time, he found it very difficult
to sterilize his solutions on account of the prevalence
in the air of bacterial spores always found on the surface of hay. From the researches of both Pasteur and
Tyndall it seems likely that the germs are not distributed uniformly throughout the atmosphere of a locality,
but form miniature clouds of floating matter separated
by intervals of pure air. For when a series of similar
vessels is exposed to the air, the separate fluids do
not all become infected at one and the same time, nor
do they all harbor the same organisms.

The question, how bacteria rise into the air, is one

*Memoire sur les corpuscles organises qui existent en suspension
dans l'atmosphere. Comptes rendus. T. 52.

of great importance, if we attribute to these beings
any role in the production of disease. It has been
shown by Naegeli* that a current of air cannot
carry off germs from a solution over which it passes.
The bacteria will not even rise out of their fluid soil,
when the air bubbles through the fluid, unless
spurting occurs. On account of these facts great
stress has been laid by Wernich† on the importance
of wetting all substances from which infective germs
might rise, in order to prevent the detachment of
the germs. Wernich found also that bacteria dried
on the surface of solid bodies, are not carried off by
currents of air, unless mechanical agitation reduces
this bacterial coating to dust. Of course any dust
light enough to remain suspended is taken up by
very faint air currents. In the case of dry porous
bodies, the detachment of adherent bacteria is more
readily produced by air permeating them with sufficient force, but is prevented ordinarily by wetting.
Still Naegeli and Buchner‡ have recently demonstrated that the porous soil of the earth will yield
germs existing in it, to ascending currents of air,
even when wet, which fact has probably quite a
bearing upon the significance of the soil in the
spreading of infectious diseases. In their experiments
a sandy soil was sterilized by heat, and then impregnated with cultivating solutions containing well-characterized forms of bacteria. On top of it were
placed glasses filled with sterilized nutritive solutions,
and the whole was covered with an inverted bell jar.

---

*Whose researches are fully quoted and corroborated by Buchner in
a lecture " On the escape of bacteria into the air," in " Vortraege
gehalten in den Sitzungen des Aerztlichen Vereins zu Munchen—Zur
Aetiologie der Infections-krankheiten. 1880, p. 293."

†Grundriss der Desinfectionslehre, 1880, p. 131 et seq.

‡Centralblatt f. d. med. Wissenschaften, No. 29, 1882.

Ascending currents of air were then started by warming the soil. The air in filtering through the pores of the sand detached bacteria and carried them up into the beakers, where the characteristic forms were found on being allowed to develop. As the air ascended through the sand a crackling noise was heard, indicative of the rupturing of minute bubbles of fluid, so that the detachment of bacteria was really due to a miniature spurting. A similar crackling noise can be observed when the surface-water changes its level in the soil of the earth, which occurrence is connected, by a large school of pathologists with changes in the sanitary condition of the locality.

LECTURE III.

Duration of Life of Bacteria.—Their Destruction by their own Products.—Antiseptic Agents.—The Struggle for Supremacy between
Different Bacteria, and between Bacteria and Animal Tissues.—
Predisposition to Parasitic Diseases.—Are there Different Kinds
of Bacteria?—The Cultivation of Bacteria.—The Variations in the
Vital Powers of Bacteria.--Mitigated Disease-germs.—Fermentations: Putrefaction. — Decomposition of Urea. — Lactic, Butyric,
Acetic, Viscous and other Fermentations.—Pigment Bacteria.—Blue
Pus: Blue Milk.—Bacteria in the Soil of the Earth.

The growth of bacteria, even in the most suitable
soil, cannot continue indefinitely. It must be remembered, that bacteria can only develop as long as they
are supplied with food, and when the soil is exhausted
their supply of food is cut off. But in reality their
growth often ceases before this theoretical limit is
attained. Almost every nutritive solution containing
bacteria regains its clearness ultimately, after the
lapse of a variable length of time. The bacteria are
deposited gradually at the bottom and all fermentative
action ceases. Examined at this time the solution may
yet be found to contain sufficient nourishment, though
all bacterial development has ceased. In some cases
the bacteria themselves are even dead, as proven by
their incapability of growing in a fresh soil. Those
species, however, which can bear spores usually pro-

duce them under these circumstances, so that the race
does not die out. In a soil in which bacteria have
ceased to multiply, it is moreover impossible to raise
another crop of the same kind on infecting the solution again with fresh bacteria or their germs. The
nutritive fluid seems to possess immunity against a
second infection.

The cause of this phenomena has been investigated
in the hope of throwing some light on the pathology
of infectious diseases. For many infectious diseases,
presumably due to the invasion of the body by microscopic parasites, have a self-limited duration comparable
to the limited growth of bacteria in a nutritive solution. Moreover, one attack of such a disease grants
the body an immunity against subsequent infection, as
we have also seen it to be the case in exhausted
culture-fluids.

Various chemists have pointed out recently, that in
the course of putrefaction several substances are
formed possessing antiseptic properties. There is
really nothing strange in this occurrence. It is quite
well known that in the case of higher animals some
of the products of their own tissue-change are poisonous, if they accumulate to an undue extent. This is
true also of some species of bacteria. Wernich* especially has called attention to the fact, that the bacteria
of putrefaction produce the very substances which,
when they accumulate sufficiently, arrest further development, or even kill their producers. Several of these
products,—for instance, indol, skatol, phenol and some
others, he subjected to the actual test, and found them
to check bacterial growth, when present to the extent
in which they actually occur in old rotten material.
He hence defends the view, that bacterial development

*Virchow's Archiv, Vol. 78, p. 51.

is ultimately arrested by the accumulation of its own products. But this is by no means true in every case. Pasteur, for instance, cultivated in chicken broth the bacteria, which cause chicken-cholera. After a few days' growth, all further development ceased. But in this case no poisonous products had accumulated; the solution was simply exhausted.

There is no proof, however, that the limited duration of certain infectious diseases depends upon either the exhaustion of the animal body with reference to some nutritive substance required by the bacteria, or upon the accumulation of bacterial products poisonous to their producers. Even if either factor were of any importance in the limitation of acute infectious diseases, it could not be supposed that it had any connection with the immunity against subsequent attacks. For in the animal economy, subject as it is to continuous tissue-change, the lack of any one ingredient of the body would soon be compensated for by its new formation, while any accumulated foreign substances would be speedily eliminated. The growth of bacteria on a dead soil cannot be compared directly with their vegetation in the living animal body. In the latter instance the parasites must compete with the animal cells, and are hence subjected to influences absent outside of the body. Any explanation intended to account for the immunity granted by the first attack of an infectious disease, must take into consideration the properties of the living animal cells and cannot be put exclusively on a chemical basis.

The development of bacteria in a suitable soil can be checked by a variety of influences which may be classified as physical, chemical, and biological.

Of the physical influences upon bacterial life none

4

are more potent than the temperature. But this topic
we have previously considered fully. It has been
stated that bacteria are also sensitive to light, their
development being checked by exposure to the sun's
rays. But the experiments do not seem to be sufficiently precise to merit further discussion. Electricity
has no direct effect upon bacteria, its destructive influence being due to the acids and alkalies formed by
electrolysis. Intense motion, however, checks bacterial
life. Howarth* found that the bacteria of putrefaction were hindered in development by shaking during
twenty-four hours the tubes in which they had been
sown, while forty-eight hours' agitation killed them.
Reinke† subsequently tried to distinguish between the
effects of a continuous motion of the fluid, and of the
sudden shocks to which the bacteria are subjected by
shaking. In order to produce these shocks at a much
more rapid rate, than can be done by mechanical
agitation, he caused waves of sound to pass through
the cultivating solution, and did thus succeed in
checking bacterial development, but could not kill
them. But then the shocks produced by sound waves
are not as violent as those due to shaking. However
suggestive these experiments may be, the research has
not been carried far enough to furnish any important
results.

The chemical influences hindering bacterial life may
relate to either the absence of necessary substances or
the presence of harmful agents. We have previously
discussed the necessity of food for bacterial life and
shown, that there are differences according to the
species which we observe. While some of the more
prevalent varieties can assimilate food offered them in

*Pflueger's Archiv f. Physiologie, Vol. 17, p. 125.
†Pflueger's Archiv, Vol. 23, p. 434.

the simplest form, others, especially the pathogenic kinds require the most elaborate animal fluids for their nutrition. Besides the nutritive substances proper there are few chemicals, the presence of which in unlimited quantity is indifferent to bacterial growth. An undue excess of even the inorganic salts, which they require normally, checks their development. Substances which can kill bacteria or arrest their growth are usually termed disinfectants or antiseptics. But these terms should not be used as loosely as they often are. Formerly, before the role of bacteria was understood any substance was called a disinfectant, provided it destroyed, or · even masked, the smell of putrefaction. Subsequently it was at least attempted to learn whether a so-called disinfectant destroyed the bacteria themselves. But the criterion at first chosen was an imperfect one. In the earlier experiments, different observers simply added the agent to be tested to bacterial fluids, and watched with the microscope the effect upon the movements. Now there are many dangerous kinds of micro-organisms, which never possess any movements, while when vital movements do exist, their arrest is by no means indicative of death. The only trustworthy criterion of the death of bacteria is the absence of their power of multiplication, when transplanted into the proper soil. By the use of appropriate methods based on this principle a more precise information as to the value of disinfectants was furnished by Buchholz*, Wernich,† and Jalan de la Croix.‡ But even these results are yet open to objections. First these authors did not distinguish between developed bacteria and their more

---

*Arch. f. experim. Pathologie, Bd. IV., p. 7.
†Virchow's Archiv, Vol. 78, p. 51.
‡Arch. f. exp. Path., B. 13, H. 3 and 4.

resistant spores, while on the other hand they did not
extend their researches to any but the common forms
of putrefaction. Koch* with his usual thoroughness
has drawn up the following program for the study of
disinfectants. It is to be learned first of all, which
is the least concentration of the substance to be
tested, requisite to check bacterial development by its
presence, without killing the bacteria. Secondly, how
much of the agent must be added in order to deprive
the developed forms permanently of their power of
reproduction, and how long must the disinfectant continue to act in order to accomplish this? Thirdly, can
the substance destroy the more resistant spores and in
what concentration? It is to be borne in mind finally
that the results thus found apply strictly only to that
kind of bacteria upon which they were obtained.
Practically, however, great differences have so far not
been found between different species, provided they are
examined at the same period of their development.

The researches of Koch have overthrown many of
our customary, but incorrect notions of disinfection.
They have shown, that it is not an easy task to kill
even the developed bacteria, while the spores defy
most so-called antiseptics. The most powerful of all
disinfectants he found in corrosive sublimate. No
other agent can as readily destroy the spores (of
bacillus anthracis and other varieties) as bichloride
of mercury, its action being instantaneous even in a
dilution of one part in five thousand, provided, of
course, there are no chemicals present, which unite
with and thus render inert the disinfectant. If not
antagonized by the presence of such interfering
substances it can permanently check bacterial growth,
as long as one part in 330,000 is present in the

---

*Mitth. aus dem Gesundheitsamt, p. 234.

solution. Next to corrosive sublimate, Koch places
bromine, iodine and chlorine. Carbolic acid, the most
common antiseptic agent, is by no means as reliable
as is usually supposed. Nothing less than a 3 per
cent. solution of it can destroy spores, requiring for
this purpose at least seven days, while a 5 per cent.
solution suffices only in from 24 to 48 hours. The
developed forms, however, it can kill quite readily
(inside of two minutes) in the strength of half of one
per cent. Its power of completely arresting bacterial
development is not manifested in any dilution of less
than 1 in 850, which suffices to check the splenic
fever bacilli, while for the common forms of putrefaction-bacteria one part in 400 to 500 is required. A
most interesting fact observed by Koch is the inert-
ness of carbolic acid when dissolved in oil. In this
form it is perfectly harmless to both spores and developed bacteria, when immersed in it in the dried state.
It can hence not be used for the disinfection of instruments, or the hands, in an oily solution. But in the
interior of wounds the carbolated oil is not so inert,
for under these circumstances some of the carbolic
acid is gradually yielded by the oil to the water
of the moist surface, in which it dissolves to form an
active solution. Dissolved in alcohol carbolic acid is
likewise wholly inert. Of other agents Koch found
very few capable of destroying spores. The only ones
that could be relied upon to accomplish this within
less than twenty-four hours were permanganate of
potassium (5 per cent.) and osmic acid (1 per cent.
sol.). A 5 per cent. solution of chloride of iron destroyed them within six days, which neither sulphate
of copper nor chloride of zinc were competent to do.
The latter agent, indeed, has been much overrated by
surgeons, according to Koch, for its presence to the

extent of half of one per cent. did not even hinder the development of the bacillus anthracis. Hydrochloric acid (2 per cent.), sulphuric acid (1 per cent.), chromic acid (1 per cent.), boracic acid (5 per cent.), tannic acid (5 per cent.), benzoic acid (concentrated) dissolved in water, as well as a host of other substances, were found inert with reference to spores. It was learned, on the other hand, by Koch, that certain substances, while not very destructive to bacteria can prevent their growth by their presence in minute quantities; for instance, allyl alcohol, one part in 167,000, mustard oil 1 in 33,000, arsenite of potassium 1 in 10,000. Researches similar to those of Koch, and on the whole confirmatory of them, have been conducted by Arloing and Thomas on the bacillus of symptomatic charbon. Since I could not obtain the original in the "Lyon Medical" I could not learn whether they distinguished strictly between the spores and the developed forms. They assign to nitrate of silver a disinfectant value, second only to corrosive sublimate. Sulphurous acid, an agent still much used for disinfection on a large scale, was found by Koch quite unreliable. Its action on spores is very feeble. While it can kill the developed forms, if present in the air to the extent of 1 per cent. (by volume) within some twenty minutes or less, it fails to penetrate into the interior of thicker masses, and its effect is therefore uncertain.

Besides the evident physical and chemical conditions which affect bacterial life, an influence is exerted also upon the growth of any bacterial variety by the co-existence of other species of micro-organisms or, in fact, any other living beings in the same soil. This influence we might term biological. Of course it should be ultimately analyzed into its physical and chemical factors,

but these we are not yet conversant with. Bacteria
like all living beings must struggle for their existence,
when forced to compete with other species. Within
certain limits different varieties can co-exist in the same
soil. Thus most rotten material contains several kinds
of bacteria. But when any one species is better
adapted to the soil than another it will soon exterminate the latter. This can be observed especially in
"pure cultures" when only one variety vegetates in
a protected soil. As soon as a different kind, of
greater reproductive power (at least under the existing
circumstances) is introduced, it will crowd the original
population out of existence. The more prevalent kinds
of bacteria found in all decomposing material are
evidently those best fitted for the struggle, as their
very prevalence shows. If hence it is desired to
cultivate in closed flasks some special kind of bacteria,
not so hardy, so to speak, as the more common species,
the least carelessness in manipulation may frustrate
the object, for if a single bacterium of a different
kind gets in by accident, it will multiply so fast as to
exterminate the others. By overlooking this fact
grave errors have been committed in the study of
alleged pure cultivations. The struggle for supremacy
between different species of bacteria explains also why
it is, that the blood of certain infectious diseases loses
its virulence, i. e. its power of producing the same
disease in other individuals on inoculation, when it is
allowed to putrefy. Thus in splenic fever and in
septicæmia the agent causing the disease has been
recognized in certain bacteria existing in the living
blood. The same blood, when rotten, is found deprived
of its special virulent properties. Its disease-breeding
bacteria have been replaced by the common micro-
organisms of putrefaction. In the case of splenic

fever blood it has been learned by Koch and by
Toussaint that the destruction of the parasites is really
caused by a deprivation of oxygen which the putrefaction-bacteria appropriate eagerly at the expense of the
pathogenic variety. For the latter are killed by the
deprivation of oxygen, no matter how produced, but
can continue their life in the presence of other
bacteria, within certain limits, if freely supplied with
that gas. In other cases it has not been learned how
one variety can crowd another out of existence,
whether it be by abstraction of the food, or oxygen,
or by the formation of products poisonous to the other
kind, or by other influences yet unknown.

When bacteria vegetate in the interior of the animal body there occurs likewise a struggle for existence
between the bacteria and the animal cells. We are
again ignorant as to the weapons of the contending
armies, we do not know yet how the warfare is carried
on between the hostile vegetable and animal cells, but
that the struggle exists is evident, and it must ter-
minate in the victory of one or the other side. The
battle won by the tissues means recovery from the
disease, while the supremacy of the invading parasites
amounts to death of the animal, or—in the more protracted cases—to perpetuation of the local disorder.
We must never lose sight of the fact that the living
animal body is not a mere "culture-flask" in which
bacteria can multiply without hindrance. If the parasites can grow at all inside of the animal system, they
can only do so by overcoming the opposition on the
part of the animal cells. But the resistance of the
animal body to the parasitic invasion varies with the
kind of bacteria and the species of animal. To illustrate this I might anticipate future remarks by pointing out that the merest trace of splenic fever bacilli

introduced into the body of a rabbit will inevitably multiply and kill the animal, while much larger numbers of the parasites can be successfully resisted by the dog. Again, while a certain kind of bacteria can readily grow in the system of the common mouse, and produce thereby the symptoms of septicæmia, they cannot be made to invade the body of a field-mouse. Such instances could easily be multiplied. But besides the differing resisting powers of different species of animals, we must recognize also variations between different individuals of the same species. Indeed, in human pathology this has always been admitted under the name "predisposition to a disease." We are all aware that apart from the influence of race and age there are individual peculiarities which render the bearer more or less likely to contract an infectious disease. The nature of this predisposition is as yet wholly unknown. Very little light has been thrown upon it by experiments on animals, mainly for the reason that the infecting material is usually employed in such massive doses, as to obliterate minor differences in the susceptibility of the victim. There is all reason to believe that in most cases the amount of infectious material producing the "natural" disease, is a mere trace, compared with the quantity employed for experimental purposes. Moreover it is not known whether the individual susceptibility varies as much in other species of animals as it does amongst mankind. Many of the shallowest arguments against the validity of the germ theory would not have been brought forth had their authors but remembered, that the pathogenic bacteria vegetating in the tissues are resisted by the animal cells, and that this resistance is variable in different cases. Our ignorance of the nature of this resistance does not justify us in overlooking it.

Throughout these lectures we have referred to different varieties of bacteria; it is now time to examine, whether the various forms met with constitute separate and distinct species, or whether all bacteria no matter what their shape are but different stages of one and the same micro-organism. There is as yet a diversity of opinion upon this subject. A certain school headed by Naegeli claims that all bacteria constitute but one species, and that the different forms are mutually convertible. On the other hand Cohn defends the view, so ably supported by Koch, that bacteria should be the generic name of a class of plants with numerous species as sharply characterized as could be expected of beings of such simple structure. But mere opinion should be of no great weight, we want facts.

It can be readily seen, that it is difficult to adduce the facts. For the proof of the correctness of one or the other view rests upon the possibility (or impossibility) of transforming one variety into another under the eyes of the observer. On account of the ubiquity of bacteria such an observation is much more difficult to make in a reliable manner than might be supposed. In order to learn whether a certain form of bacteria represents a distinct species we must cultivate it, as we would any higher plant, in different soils and under different circumstances. But every time the flask is opened in which this is done and every time we transfer a drop to a new flask we run the risk of the accidental introduction of other germs from the air, even if we purify our instruments and vessels scrupulously. The crop therefore which we raise may not be at all derived from the stock we have sown. Hence it is very difficult to maintain the purity of a successive series of cultures in flasks. This difficulty is not diminished, though the occurrence of an impurity can be more readily detected, if we take such a small quantity of the cultivating solution, that the whole culture can be surveyed under the microscope. This can be done by placing a single drop on the under surface of a cover-glass resting upon a hollow glass slide, or supported by a ring of parafine upon an ordinary slide. By means of this method the growth of bacteria can be watched continuously, or at intervals, and the entrance of any foreign species detected speedily. This method, however, is applicable only to those forms presenting a characteristic appearance easily recognized. A decided improvement for the maintenance of a culture in a state of purity, has lately been introduced by Koch. This consists in the use of a *solid* soil. A solution of gelatine, about 3 per cent. in strength, is allowed to congeal in watch glasses, or in the form of flat drops simply on a slide. It must contain an addition of meat extract, blood serum, vegetable infusions, or some other nutritive substances. It is to be sterilized previously by repeated heating according to the method of Tyndall. A temperature of 58° C. cannot be surpassed if serum is used, without coagulating the latter. Moreover this suffices if repeated for about an hour at a time. The bacteria are planted on this solid soil by scratching it with a needle dipped into the material from which the bacteria are to be derived. The great advantage of this method is the absence of currents in the soil. The progeny of each single bacterium cannot be carried hither and thither as would be the case in fluids, but remains collected around the centre, where the parent cell was implanted. This is true of the bacteria we sow as well as of the germs which get in accidentally. The entrance of foreign bacteria coming from the air we cannot prevent altogether, but the crop which they engender does not get mixed with the bacteria under observation. It extends more or less rapidly from the spot where the foreign germs settled, but does not invade the whole soil. Experience has shown, that different bacteria growing on such a solid soil can be distinguished by the different forms of colonies which they produce, and by the manner in which the growth extends. According to the kind under observation the growth appears in the form of larger or smaller globules, arborescent projections, flat scums, or simply diffused masses radiating from the furrow of implantation, with or without liquefaction of the soil. Hence with a low power of the microscope, or even with the naked eye any impurity of the culture due to foreign germs can be detected in time, and the desired purity be maintained by transferring a trace from the intact portion to a fresh sterilized soil. Impregnated gelatine is not the only available solid soil, though it possesses the special advantage of transparency. Many of the more prevalent forms can grow on the surface of a slice of a boiled potato. In fact observations on this substratum suggested to Koch the advantage of a solid soil. A drawback to the gelatine soil is its low melting point, viz: 28° C. In my own experience most of the grades to be had in commerce here became fluid at even a lower temperature in spite of accurate neutralization of any trace of acidity present. In order to obviate this difficulty Koch has lately used solidified blood serum. The blood is allowed to clot in a purified vessel, and after standing twenty-four hours in a cool place the serum is drained off. This is then heated to 58° C. an hour at a time during several successive days in order to sterilize it, hereupon it is transferred into suitable vessels and converted into an amber-like gelatinous solid mass by heating it up to 65° C. This transparent soil offers the best possible nutrition to pathogenic bacteria, and unlike gelatine does not melt on warming.

On taking a historical review of the evidence brought forth in favor of either the mutability, or stability, of bacterial species, we will find that the former view has been steadily losing ground. As the methods of cultivation became more reliable and their sources of error were better understood, it had to be admitted that in most cases the alleged transformation of one kind into another was simply the substitution of accidentally admitted germs for the original stock. Some fifteen years ago Hallier, one of the pioneers in bacterial morphology claimed that mould-fungi, yeast cells, and bacteria were but different stages of one and the same plant. But it was soon shown by competent botanists, that his methods were untrust-worthy.

At the present time no one claims that bacteria can ever change into any other form of plants. That superstition has been settled long ago and in a very positive manner. But Naegeli and his adherents still think that a given form of bacteria can change its appearance and physiological properties, in fact be converted into another variety, when placed under altered circumstances. With the exception, however, of one doubtful observation by Buchner there remains no proof in favor of that view. So far as all trust-worthy observation goes, every bacterial species retains all its morphological characteristics, no matter in what soil it grows, if it grows at all. A bacillus never changes into a micrococcus, nor the latter into a spirillum. Even minor points of shape remain constant.

Rod-shaped bacteria possessing a square end do not round off their extremity on growing in another medium, and vice versa. Likewise the peculiar form in which the growth extends on solid soil, remains the same, no matter how often the species is transplanted. The chemical and vital properties likewise are peculiar to each bacterial variety. The ꞌ micro-organism which causes lactic acid fermentation cannot start the putrefaction of albumen, or ferment glycerine. The bacillus producing splenic fever is not the cause of any other disease and the bacteria of septicæmia do not produce tuberculosis or other affections.

This question of the mutability or stability of bacterial forms is evidently one of great importance. Were it possible, for instance, to change harmless bacteria of putrefaction into potent disease germs, through influences which occur in nature, there would be little hope of ever eradicating any infectious disease. But, I must repeat, all evidence, when carefully weighed, points towards the permanency of the separate bacterial species. Of course the question cannot be decided any other way but by experiment; it would be unscientific to assume on theoretical grounds that the conversion of one form into another can never be realized. But the fact is, that this has not been accomplished as yet under any conditions tested, and we must therefore recognize a large. number of separate and distinct species of bacteria as permanent varieties in the present state of our science. The validity of certain experiments to the contrary we shall discuss under the head of splenic fever.

Pasteur, whose stronghold is evidently not microscopical morphology, suggested some time since that the classification of bacteria should be physiological rather than anatomical. He pointed out that different

species, which he could not distinguish from each
other with the microscope, still possessed different
vital properties. Of micro-organisms, apparently alike
in form, some produce different fermentations; others
can cause various diseases. His criterion of a species
therefore was not merely the form, but rather the
chemical or vital test. But his own later researches
have shown that this system of classification is not
tenable. For he himself has made the important
discovery that the properties of a given species may
vary in degree with different circumstances, and that
this altered vital power is then transmitted to the
succeeding generations. The first instance in which
he showed this variability of the vital power of a
species was in the case of the parasites producing
chicken-cholera. These micrococci after once entering
the body of a fowl multiply there to an unlimited
extent, and with rare exceptions destroy their host's
life. The parasites could be cultivated in chicken-
broth, in which their further growth ceased after
some four or five days. They retained their original
virulence,—i. e. their power of struggling victoriously
with the tissues of the fowl—indefinitely, if they were
transferred to a fresh soil from time to time. But
when they were allowed to remain for months in the
same flask, their vital power was gradually reduced.
Samples taken from the flask at successive intervals
were found less and less poisonous to the animal.
The older the crop of parasites the less vigorous was
their growth in the animal body, and the milder the
disease to which they gave rise. About nine months'
sojourn in the unchanged medium deprived these
bacteria of their ability to multiply at all in the
animal body, though they could still grow in a fresh
cultivating solution. A still longer sojourn in the

same flask without change of soil, killed them.
Pasteur attributes the enfeebling of the bacterial
vitality to the influence of the oxygen. For when
the flasks were hermetically closed the lapse of time
alone did not reduce the bacterial power of reproduction or their virulence to animals. A further
point of capital importance discovered by Pasteur is
the fact, that the altered degree of virulence is transmitted unchanged through the successive generations,
when the bacteria thus enfeebled are cultivated in
a fresh soil. He succeeded thus in transforming one
variety of bacteria into another, if we take the physiological properties as the criterion of a variety. If
on the other hand we take the more correct standpoint of characterizing a species by its morphology,
these researches teach us that the vital power of a
bacterial variety, i. e. the ability to struggle for its
existence against the opposition of other living cells,
can be permanently altered. Pasteur has since shown
the same to be true of the splenic fever bacilli, and,
he claims, also of other pathogenic bacteria.
Whether the power of bacteria to start certain
fermentations can be permanently altered by the
mode of cultivation has not been much investigated.
I can find but a single statement by Fitz, who
claims that a certain bacillus producing the butyric
fermentation of glycerine loses this property by
successive cultivation at 45° C., or by raising several
generations in a solution of meat extract having a
large surface exposed to the air. In the case of
some disease germs it has been further shown by
some French observers (Toussaint, Chauveau), that
any temporary influences which, if persistent, would
destroy the bacteria, reduce permanently their power
of multiplying in and harming the animal body.

The evidence of clinical medicine, which, it must be admitted, can only be suggestive, and never as positive as experimental proof, supports the views here presented. The study of contagious diseases leads to the inference that disease germs are distinct and separate species, but that their virulence can vary. The infection from a small-pox patient, or a case of scarlet fever, or measles, produces only the original infection and never any other disease, but the severity of an epidemic varies a great deal in different years.

A satisfactory study of the role of bacteria can only be undertaken from the standpoint thus presented, viz: that there are numerous species differing from each other by their structure, shape, mode of growth and properties. If we do not admit—at least provisionally—the stability of each species, we will have no guiding thread to follow through the confusion of observations. Even should further research show, that different varieties of bacteria can be transformed into each other under conditions with which we are not yet acquainted, it would not invalidate our knowledge regarding any one species. From this point of view the balance of our studies ought logically to be devoted to the natural history of each separate species of bacteria. But our information is as yet too incomplete to permit of such a systematic arrangement. It will be more convenient to discuss the various occurrences in which bacteria are known to be concerned, beginning with fermentations, and then passing in review the various diseases, the parasitic origin of which is either proven or suspected.

Fermentation and putrefaction have been defined above as processes of decomposition, in which complex molecules are split up into simpler ones. It should

now be added that these chemical changes are due to
the life-work of micro-organisms.   It is characteristic
of them, that the mass of living cells accomplishing
the change may be very small, when compared with
the amount of material transformed.   In what manner
the micro-organisms affect the chemical ·changes is but
imperfectly known.   It has been shown in some
instances, that they form soluble substances termed
ferments, which produce the chemical changes by
themselves, independent of the bacteria, which generated the ferment.   These ferments can also act when
present in remarkably small quantities, even after the
living cells producing them have been removed.   But
a non-living soluble ferment can never multiply or
reproduce itself.   That faculty is the exclusive privi-
lege of living beings.   In many fermentations, however,
no soluble ferments have ever been detected and the
chemical changes in these cases can only occur in
the interior of the living cells.   The energy of a
fermentative process, is greatest at the temperature
most favorable to the life of the species of micro-
organisms concerned.

The most common fermentative process in nature is
the decomposition, or rotting, of complex nitrogenous
material, like albuminoids, gelatine and the allied vegetable substances.   It occurs invariably, when such
substances are exposed to the air under proper conditions of moisture and temperature, and in the absence
of antiseptic agents.   Hence ordinarily all animal and
vegetable refuse rots.   The successive chemical stages
of the putrefactive change have as yet been incom-
pletely traced.   The changes which albumen undergoes
resemble at first the process of digestion.   It is converted into soluble forms partly peptone, and then split
up into leucin and tyrosin.   Subsequently numerous

volatile fatty acids, and various polyatomic alcohols
(phenol, skatol, indol) appear as well as a host of
other substances in traces. Amongst them are a
variety of poisonous agents, especially some alkaloids
(ptomaines). At last the bulk of these derivatives is
converted into the simplest chemical forms (partly by
oxydation), viz.: ammonia, carbonic acid, water, sulphuretted hydrogen (and phosphoretted hydrogen). The
most constant bacterial form met with in putrefaction
is the bacterium termo. It consists of rods two to
three micromillimeters in length, one-fifth to one-half
as thick, often in pairs, sometimes in zoogloea masses.
It is freely mobile, possessing a most delicate flagellum
at either end. It is not known to form spores. It is
distinctly aerobic, requiring oxygen for its growth and
movements. Pasteur, who does not admit that aerobic
bacteria can cause fermentation, claims that the bacterium termo, living at the surface of rotting material,
merely oxydizes the derivatives, but does not produce
the original decomposition. Nencki, who also defends
this view, seeks the cause of the original decomposition principally in different micrococci living in the
depth of the material. The latter can continue their
work in the absence of oxygen when the bacterium
termo disappears. Usually there are also different
forms of larger bacilli present, amongst them often
the kind known as the hay bacillus, or the bacillus
subtilis. This micro-organism, one of the most common in nature, is found dried on the surface of hay
and many grains. It consists of delicate rods with
flagella either in separate segments some two to six
micromillimeters in length, or—especially when not
shaken—in the form of very long undivided threads.
On account of the resisting power of its spores it is
very apt to appear or rather to persist in fluids which

have been boiled. Its presence has therefore been a
stumbling-block to many a champion of spontaneous
generation. It cannot live without oxygen, and forms
hence a membrane-like scum on the surface of the
fluids in which it grows, without rendering them turbid in the depth. It cannot cause rotting by itself.
But other bacilli of different forms and different properties are almost always met with in rotting material,
besides the micrococci above mentioned. Putrid refuse
presents really an extensive flora of microscopic beings.
Hence, besides the putrefaction bacteria proper, it may
harbor disease germs, though they are not always
present.

A second form of fermentation of nitrogenous
material of special medical interest is the transformation of urea into carbonate of ammonia. Urine when
exposed to the air, especially in the vicinity of barns
and closets, is apt to become ammoniacal. This change
is due to the presence of the micrococcus ureæ. If
this micrococcus be excluded the urine does not turn
alkaline, although other bacteria may cause rotting.
Recent researches by Jaksch* have shown that this
bacterium appears at first in the form of rods two to
three micromillimeters in length by one half a micromillimeter in width, which speedily segment and in
the course of forty-eight hours form micrococci-like
granules — in chains. Gradually these micrococci
assume the zoogloea form, sink to the bottom, and after
the lapse of some four or six weeks die, unless transferred to a fresh soil. Their life and activity requires
the presence of oxygen. They thrive best at a
temperature of 30° to 33° C., and are killed by 60° C.
Jaksch presents some interesting observations on their
nutrition. Any artificial solution intended to nourish

*Zeitschrift f. physiologische Chemie. Bd. V., p. 395.

them, must contain of inorganic salts potassium and
magnesium in the form of phosphate and sulphate.
They cannot develop in the absence of any one of
these elements. They require besides some source of
nitrogen and carbon, which latter element they cannot
obtain from urea alone. Urea is transformed by them
into bicarbonate of ammonium by union with two
molecules of water. This chemical change is effected
by means of a soluble ferment secreted by these
bacteria, which latter can be isolated by precipitation
with alcohol. In some diseases of the bladder, and
especially in paralysis of that organ from spinal
disease, the urine is ammoniacal when freshly voided.
In such instances the micrococcus ureæ is always
present in the bladder, and has always been introduced from without. The most common way of
introduction is evidently the use of impure catheters
or sounds. In reply to doubts of the truth of this
statement, Pasteur challenged the French Academy of
Medicine in 1877 to produce a case of ammoniacal
urine in which he could not show the presence of
these bacteria, but this was never done. Possibly the
bacteria may creep into the bladder by growth
through the urethra, when this channel is kept filled
with the dribbling urine, but this is not yet certain.
In the healthy bladder the micrococcus ureæ cannot
find the conditions requisite for its continued vegetation. As was shown by Feltz and Ritter, the injection
of these bacteria into the healthy bladders of dogs is
soon followed by their elimination.

The hydrocarbons can undergo a variety of fermentations. Starch can be attacked by bacterium termo,
but, as Wortmann* has shown, only when there is no
other source of carbon available. In that case a fer-

*Zeitschrift f. physiologische Chemie. Bd. VI., p. 287.

ment-like diastase is secreted, which transforms the starch into sugar. The sugar is consumed by the bacteria as fast as it is formed.

The fermentation of sugar into alcohol is not due to bacteria, but is ordinarily the work of the yeast plant. The same change can also be accomplished by various mould fungi, even the . common penicillium, when submerged in the saccharine solution, so as to be deprived of oxygen. As far as we know, no bacteria can produce this fermentation.

The lactic acid fermentation of sugars is produced by a certain species of bacteria, in the form of micrococci in chains or pairs. (Lister* and Meyer.†) The size seems to be somewhat variable. This micro-organism gets into the milk, when freshly drawn, either from the teats or from the utensils used. It seems very difficult to exclude this micro-organism on collecting milk. Moreover it is not readily killed by heat, as it can certainly withstand the boiling temperature for a short time, according to Pasteur and others. Yet it is not known whether it exists in the form of spores; indeed its morphology has been but imperfectly investigated. It changes milk sugar, grape sugar and allied varieties into lactic acid, but this transformation does not continue long unless alkalies are present to neutralize the acid as fast as it is formed. For these bacteria are very sensitive to any excess of acid. It is claimed that they are anærobic. Their presence is the cause of the souring of milk. Of course the higher the temperature of the season the quicker this change occurs. In what manner the occurrence of a thunder shower can affect the rapidity of this process—if it really does so—has never been investigated.

---

*Transactions of the London Pathological Society, 1878.
†Maly's Jahresbericht f. Thierchemie, 1881. p. 468.

The fermentation of lactic acid into butyric acid is also due to the life-work of bacteria. This species consists of large rods, often in the form of lengthy chains, endowed with slow serpentine movements, and capable of growing and acting only in the absence of free oxygen (Pasteur).

There occurs, furthermore, a viscous or ropy fermentation of sugars found at times both in wines and milk. The sugar is thereby transformed into a gum-like substance, giving the solution a ropy consistency. The cause of this change is a large micrococcus, usually in the form of chains.*

The acetic acid fermentation of alcohol is usually produced by a species of large micrococci (one to three micromillimeters in diameter) which form a dense scum on the surface of the alcoholic liquid. The oxydation of alcohol into acetic acid can be accomplished also by some other varieties, while a different species, not yet closely studied, can oxydize the alcohol completely into carbonic acid and water. All these forms require the presence of oxygen and are checked in their action by too great a concentration of the alcohol. Unlike other bacterial species, they can thrive in an acid medium.

Some interesting fermentations involving glycerine have been studied by Fitz in several communications made to the German Chemical Society (since 1876). In a cultivating solution containing three per cent. of glycerine he observed transformation of the latter into ethyl alcohol (at least in part) from the action of a rod-shaped bacterium, which he obtained by washing the surface of hay. (Buchner has lately denied, however, that this is the common bacillus subtilis.) This fermentation is a very slow one. A quicker fermenta-

---

*Pasteur, also Schmidt-Muhlheim. Pflueger's Archiv. f. d. ges. Physiologie. Bd. 27, p. 490.

tion of glycerine resulting in the formation of butyric acid, butyl-alcohol, and other products was obtained by the agency of another bacillus larger than the former, but derived like it from the surface of hay.

Certain fermentations result in the appearance of colored products. The best known instance of this kind is the life-work of the micrococcus prodigiosus. This bacterium grows readily on the surface of certain solid soils, like potato slices, bread, and other victuals, and gives rise to a nearly blood-red scum. This singular growth of blood-like patches, which may infest a locality like an epidemic, has often attracted popular attention, and has formerly started many a superstition. The phenomenon, however, is simply due to the vegetation of a micrococcus, colorless by itself, but producing a red pigment insoluble in water and having some chemical resemblance to aniline colors. Usually this micrococcus is crowded out after a few days' vegetation by an invasion of the same soil by other bacteria of putrefaction, which also destroy the pigment formed. It was observed in Cohn's laboratory that continued experimentation with this micro-organism caused such a diffusion of the germs (dried cocci or spores?) throughout the air, that any suitable soil became invariably affected, when exposed to the atmospheric dust. Various other pigment bacteria have been studied by Schroeter* and Cohn.† Quite a variety of pigments could thus be obtained by the action of different micro-organisms. In these instances the stability of the bacterial species can be readily demonstrated even without the microscope. For each species produces only its own peculiar pigment, if the soil permits the formation of the latter, and never any other.

---

*Cohn's Beitraege z. Biologie d. Pflanzen, Bd. I., H.-II, p. 109.
†Idem, p. 151.

The blue coloration of pus sometimes observed on surgical dressings is also the product of bacterial action. This form consists of very thin elliptic rods about 1 to 1.8 micromillimeters in length, partly united in pairs. The pigment was found by Fitz to resemble litmus in its chemical behavior. It is originally colorless, but under the influence of the atmospheric oxygen it turns blue. Under some circumstances the presence of this same species stains the pus yellow. According to surgical experience the presence of these parasites in wounds is of no special importance.

Very singular observations have been made by Neelsen* on the bacteria which cause the epidemics of "blue milk" in dairies. This fermentation, resulting in the production of a soluble blue pigment is the work of short mobile bacilli vegetating in the milk. They are not known to render the milk injurious. After a few days' growth (by fission) they change their shape and form chains of shorter segments, which do not undergo further change until transferred into a fresh soil. Since these short, biscuit-shaped segments do not possess any great resisting power to damaging influences, Neelsen does not consider them true spores, but compares them to the "gonidia" of higher fungi. But true spores were observed, when these bacteria (or their gonidia) were sown in Cohn's cultivating solution. The growth of the bacteria in this soil was not attended by the formation of any pigments. But when an addition of lactate of ammonia was made to Cohn's solution the blue pigment was produced. The shape, however, of the plant was entirely altered in this solution, in which it assumed the appearance of micrococci in zooglœa masses. Neelsen claims that this strange metamorphosis is normal to this species when planted in

*Beitr. z. Biologie d. Pflanzen, Bd. III. Heft II., p. 187.

different soils, for he could always produce the original
form of the bacterium by transplanting it back to milk.
These interesting observations, however, need confirmation.

The life-work of certain bacteria reveals itself by a
phosphorescence of the vegetation. Sometimes animal
refuse, especially salt-water fish, is covered with a slimy
coat emitting a feeble glow in the dark. In a specimen of meat of this kind Lassar found the cause to
be the growth of a micrococcus on the surface.

The above list includes the fermentations best known,
but by no means all the instances of chemical changes,
owing to the presence of bacteria. It shows, however,
the important role played by these minute beings in
the household of nature. Their significance is the
more apparent, when we take into consideration that
they are not only concerned in so many chemical processes on the surface of the globe, but also in a
continuous series of changes occurring in the soil of
the earth. The form in which the nitrogen exists in
the soil undergoes changes, and with it the value of
the soil for agricultural purposes. Schloesing and
Muntz showed some time ago that the oxydation of
ammonia salts and other nitrogenous compounds into
the form of nitrates is the work of living bacteria.
Within the last year various communications have been
made to the French Academy by other observers to
prove that there occurs likewise a change in the other
direction, viz.: the reduction of nitrates to a less oxy-
dized form. This process is also due to the life-work
of bacteria.

LECTURE IV.

Bacteria on the Surface of the Animal Body and in the Digestive Canal.—Their Work in Digestion.—Germs in the Healthy Tissues. —The Research for Pathogenic Bacteria.—Microscopic Detection, Cultivation and Inoculation of Germs.—Charbon.—Its Parasites and their Mode of Producing and Spreading the Disease.—Protective Vaccination with Mitigated Germs.—The Germicide Treatment.—Chicken-cholera.

The prevalence of bacteria, in the vegetating condition and dried in suspension in the air, evidently brings them into contact with the animal body. They exist, usually in a dried state, on the surface of the skin and hair, and cannot be removed entirely by washing. If secretions occur in which they can vegetate, bacterial life and activity are soon manifested. Thus—as Thin has shown—bacteria cause the foul odor of bad-smelling feet by their decomposition of the sweat, and the persistence of this annoyance is due to their vegetation in the ducts of the cutaneous glands. With every breath we take, bacteria are deposited upon the respiratory surfaces. The expired air seems to be filtered mainly in the narrow pulmonary spaces, and thereby loses the most of the particles it contained in suspension. Tyndall has shown that the last portion of the exhaled breath does not scatter light and is hence optically pure. Gunning has lately

attempted to prove the purity of the expired air in
another manner. On allowing it to bubble through a
sterilized cultivating solution he obtained no infection
of the fluid. But from the negative results in similar
experiments by others with common air, I am inclined
to doubt the reliability of this method. Air in bub-
bling through fluids does not probably yield its dust
readily to them. With every morsel of food we consume, bacteria are carried into the digestive canal,
where they find the conditions present required for
their growth, viz.: food, moisture and the proper heat.
In the mouth some forms or other are always met
with, the most common one being the Leptothrix buccalis, a chain of short thick segments. Frequently
also a delicate spirillum with many convolutions occurs
on the surface of the teeth. Sternberg has found a
micrococcus in the saliva of some healthy people which
can produce septicæmia in rabbits.

In the stomach bacterial activity is normally checked
by the acid of the gastric juice, although this is
hardly of sufficient strength to kill all forms. When
the secretion of the acid ceases during a disease, lactic
and butyric acid fermentations and perhaps other bacterial processes do occur. In the intestines, however,
where the reaction is either alkaline or only faintly
acid, bacteria thrive luxuriously. Their vegetation is
so rank, that the normal fæces, if not augmented in
bulk by undigested remnants of food, may consist
almost entirely of bacteria. Nothnagel,* who has lately
re-examined this question, finds in the stools quite a
variety of forms of both micrococci and bacilli. Their
existence in the intestines is not a morbid occurrence;
it is normal and—in my opinion—explains one of the
puzzles in the physiology of digestion. Busch and

---

*Zeitschrift f. klinische Medicin, Bd. 3, p. 275.

others who have had the chance to investigate cases
of intestinal fistula in man or in animals have found,
that many solid food substances are absorbed in the
intestines without the aid of gastric or pancreatic juice.
On the other hand examination of the intestinal juice
proper shows that it has but feeble digestive properties.
It is likely that the discrepancies between the different
observers, who studied intestinal digestion in and outside of the intestines, are due to overlooking the
putrefactive processes which normally occur in the
intestines. Certainly the changes which are observed
in artificial digestion in flasks do not comprise all
those found in the intestinal canal. Normal digestion
is evidently complicated by putrefaction. The presence
of these bacterial parasites in the intestinal canal is
not at all a damage, but it seems a benefit to the
animal, for they evidently supplement the action of
the digestive juices. In the case of one substance at
least — cellulose — the digestion in the intestinal tract
of herbivora is entirely the work of bacteria.

In the instances so far considered the bacteria exist
only on the surface—be it external or internal—of the
body. But a different question, and one of capital
importance with relation to the germ theory is: do
bacteria, or their germs exist in the *interior* of a
healthy organism, in the blood or in the tissues
themselves?

The microscope cannot detect them in the healthy
blood and tissues even with the aid of the most delicate staining methods, but this would be insufficient
evidence, if their number is very limited. The question can be only decided by the cultivation of any
pre-existing germs with the exclusion of any coming
from the outside. Numerous such experiments have
been made. Van der Brock, Pasteur, Lister and others

all agree that living blood received in purified vessels
with antiseptic precautions will not putrefy. Putrefactive bacteria do not pre-exist in the living blood
vessels. Recently Zweifel* has denied the accuracy of
this statement and claimed that the germs which do
pre-exist are prevented from developing by the oxygen
of the arterial blood. For, when he removed the
oxygen, putrefaction set in, and he claims even to
have seen micrococci (though without putrefaction) in
the arterial blood on standing in closed vessels. But
his work does not bear such a stamp of accuracy as
to entitle it to much faith. To start with, he overlooks the fact that the oxygen of the shed blood disappears pretty soon, under any circumstances, while
in his attempts to pump out the gases of the blood
he undoubtedly infected it with germs from without.
Moreover, he did not prove, that the granules which
he saw in the blood were really micrococci and not
the detritus of white blood-corpuscles.

That the normal urine does not decompose, when
protected against outside germs has been found by all
observers. In the case of the milk it has been
learned by Lister, Cheyne, and Meissner that it
contains originally no germs, but that it is difficult to
collect it without introducing lactic acid bacteria from
the teats.

Whether bacteria pre-exist in the solid tissues, Billroth attempted to decide by cutting pieces out of the
body and throwing them into melted parafine, which
was intended to exclude foreign germs. In all his
experiments putrefaction occurred. These observations
have since been repeated by many others, but with
variable results. Although various careful observers,
for instance, Nencki and Giacosa,† who worked appar-

*Zeitschrift f. phys. Chemie. Vol. VI., p. 386.
†Journal f. pract. Chemie, Vol. 20, p. 34. 1879.

ently with all the precautions of antiseptic surgery, have found that they could not preserve tissues in their fresh state without decomposition, still it must now be admitted that the germs of putrefaction do not pre-exist in the healthy living body. For other experimenters *have* succeeded in preserving the fresh tissues unaltered, by the exclusion of germs from without. Chiene and Ewarts placed various extirpated organs partly into carbolated gauze, partly into flasks previously purified by heat, and found them pure after the lapse of many days, and without the presence of bacteria. But the most extensive research on this topic seems to have been conducted by Meissner, as reported by Rosenbach.* Since his object was to learn whether germs existed in living tissues, he avoided the use of any antiseptic agents which could destroy them, but observed the greatest care in transferring his pieces from the animal just killed to flasks previously heated. By working in a clean room, using only instruments just heated, manipulating with the utmost quickness and delicacy, he succeeded in keeping his specimens free from putrefaction in the majority of instances. A most important lesson which his experiments taught, and which serves to explain the contrary results of other observers, is the fact that with increasing practice the number of failures became less, and he could at last preserve almost every specimen. The weight of evidence is pretty conclusive, therefore, that the living healthy animal does not harbor bacteria in its tissues.

Moreover, it has been shown that the bacteria of putrefaction are soon destroyed or eliminated if purposely introduced into the animal system. If they

*Zeitschrift f. Chirurgie, Vol. XIII, p. 344.

be injected into the blood, and the animal does not
die from the poisonous effects of some of the products
of putrefaction, the blood rids itself speedily of these
micro-organisms. If drawn, after the lapse of a few
hours, and received in purified vessels it remains free
from putrefaction, showing that no germs are left in
it (Cheyne). In the struggle with the animal cells
the common bacteria of putrefaction are overcome.
But this is not true of all bacterial varieties. There
are numerous micro-organisms, which find the conditions met with in the animal system suitable to their
existence, and can lead a parasitic life in the midst
of the tissues. But this vegetation of parasites in
the interior of the animal body is not a normal
occurrence as far as the latter is concerned; some
disturbance or other is always created thereby, and
such parasitic bacteria constitute true disease germs.

The bacterial origin of a disease can only be
proven by the following observations. First, a characteristic bacterial species must always be found associated with the disease, and to an extent corresponding to the nature and degree of the disease.
Secondly, it must be shown that the same disease can
be reproduced in susceptible beings by means of the
isolated parasites, freed from all animal matter 'or
poisons. It is not an easy matter to furnish these
proofs in the case of any disease; it requires
thorough familiarity with the methods, and a critical
spirit. In order to demonstrate the bacteria in the
tissues, staining methods must be resorted to. It is
only when the parasites form large colonies, especially
in the interior of the vessels, that they can be seen
by simply clearing the section with acetic acid or
alkalies. For staining purposes the different aniline
colors must be tested, since different bacteria react

differently to such colors. Special complications in the staining process have been found necessary in the case of the bacilli of leprosy and of tuberculosis. Probably there exist yet many pathogenic varieties which we have not seen on account of the inability to stain them with present means. ' In the examination of stained sections diffuse illumination by means of an appropriate condensor, is absolutely indispensable. Not all the colored particles seen are bacteria. Careless manipulation may give rise to precipitates. The granules found in many cells, in white blood-corpuscles, and especially in the plasma cells of Ehrlich, resemble micrococci. The distinction between micrococci and other colored granules is absolute only, when by reason of their growth they are found in regularly arranged colonies. Of course the specimens should be taken either from the living subject or very soon after death, in order not to be misled by the bacteria of putrefaction invading the cadaver. Finally the absence of bacteria must not be inferred, when they are sought for and not found in an improper place, for instance the blood in some local disease, or some organ affected only indirectly.

The only mode of isolating parasitic bacteria from the animal tissues is by means of cultivation of the former in a proper soil. The animal cells which we transfer with them to the soil die at once, while any chemical poisons associated with them cannot multiply like the living bacteria themselves. The implantation of a trace of the first crop in a fresh soil, and a few repetitions of this procedure, dilute any foreign matter adhering to the bacteria to such an extent as to practically eliminate it. It is evidently of vital importance, that the bacteria sown should be the real parasites, and not merely accidental associates. It is,

hence, best to take the matter to be cultivated from
the interior of the body, in preference to secretions on
the surface, exposed to the germs of the air. A
successful cultivation requires evidently, that the soil
should be appropriate to the species examined. Most
pathogenic bacteria cannot thrive as readily as the
germs of putrefaction on a soil as simple as Pasteur's
or Cohn's solution. In many cases they require a
nourishing fluid closely resembling the blood itself.
The successful cultivation of an isolated species
without the unwelcome admixture of other germs is
much facilitated by the employment of a solid soil
after the fashion of Koch.

The proof of a parasitic origin of a disease is only
complete, when the same disease can be reproduced by
inoculation with the cultivated bacteria. It is not
sufficient that the animal gets sick in consequence of
the inoculation; it must be affected with the original
disease in question. A species of animals which can
not take a certain disease can, therefore, not be used to
prove the origin of that disorder. In this respect there
are wide differences in different animals. Splenic fever,
so fatal to herbivora, cannot be easily produced in car-
nivora, and—it seems—never in the pig. A form of
septicæmia common to the house-mouse cannot attack
the field-mouse. Different species of animals constitute
different soils for the bacterial parasites, and it is self-
evident that a plant cannot grow in all soils. Some
parasitic diseases of mankind cannot be transferred to
any animal yet employed, for instance, gonorrhœa.
Again, in other cases, the same parasite produces a
different reaction in different animals. The bacteria
which give septicæmia to mice cause in rabbits but a
local inflammation comparable to erysipelas. The susceptibility of an animal species to a certain disease is

sometimes a question of the quantity of disease germs. Both anthrax and tuberculosis are not readily communicated to dogs, except a certain number of the pathogenic germs be employed, while perhaps a single germ suffices for the invasion of the body of a rabbit. Probably the number of disease germs is of importance also with reference to the variable individual susceptibility, especially in the natural infection, when undoubtedly much smaller quantities of germs enter the system than in experimental inoculation. The success of an inoculation with bacteria may depend also on the purity of the culture. For when we employ, instead of the isolated parasites, a mixture of different bacteria the pathogenic variety may be overpowered by its accidental associates, which by themselves are perhaps harmless to the animal body. Finally, the inoculation must be made in the proper place in order to succeed. Various germs can not enter with equal facility through all the gates of the organism. Thus the bacillus of malignant œdema can gain a foothold only in deep wounds and not in mere abrasions of the skin. The bacilli of symptomatic charbon are fatal when put under the skin, but nearly harmless when injected into the blood-vessels. Hence false conclusions should not be drawn when an improper mode of inoculation fails to lodge the parasites in the animal body. As an instance of such an error I might mention the experiments of Wolff, who concluded that bacteria were harmless to wounds, because abrasions in the skin of animals healed just as well, when covered with rotten material containing bacteria. The very fact that these wounds healed kindly ordinarily, although exposed to the germs of the air, dust, and material with which the animals come in contact, shows that the open surface of a wound does not grant germs a ready entrance into the system, at least in rabbits or guinea

pigs. Moreover, there is a real difference between the
course of such wounds, as are unavoidably or intentionally
exposed to bacteria, and those which are properly protected against them, which fact Wolff overlooked.

Having thus discussed what requirements must be
insisted upon in order to admit the bacterial origin of
any one disease, let us now pass in review the list of
diseases, to which such research has been applied. It
will be most convenient to begin with those instances
which have been investigated more satisfactorily than
others.

ANTHRAX.

The first and best known instance of a disease definitely traced to the invasion of the body by vegetable
parasites is splenic fever, also called anthrax, charbon,
or—in the localized form usually seen in man,—malignant pustule. It is a disease occurring principally in
cattle and sheep, but is inoculable in most domestic
animals.

In this disease rod-shaped bacteria were found in
the blood, originally by Rayer and Davaine in 1850,
and later independently of them by Pollender (1855) and
Brauell (1857). Their vegetable nature was assumed,
but not proven. Delafond (1860) seems to have been
the first to suspect these bodies as the cause of the
disease. Subsequently Davaine (1863) rendered this
suspicion extremely probable, by showing that they
were always present in the blood of this disease, that
splenic fever could only be produced by inoculation
with material containing them, and that those influences which destroyed the "bacteridia" as he called
them, deprived the blood of its special virulence.

The absolute proof of their importance, viz.: the
production of the disease by means of the isolated

bacteria, has since been furnished by Koch and repeated by Pasteur and many others.

As seen in the blood of an affected animal the
bacillus anthracis consists of slender rods having a
length of upwards of about three micromillimeters
and dividing usually into segments, when they exceed
six micromillimeters. Since the segmentation is not
visible except on staining, we find in the fresh specimen some few filaments, apparently undivided, as long
as twenty micromillimeters. Its width, as Huber* has
shown, varies somewhat according to the species of
animal in which it lives—about 1 to 1.3 micromillimeters. Its ends are square, or even slightly concave
—as seen when two segments adhere before separation,—which shape characterizes this bacillus. It has
no flagella and is motionless (except immediately
after germination). As long as it grows in the bodies
of living animals it assumes no other shape but the
one described, and multiplies only by fission. But
when cultivated outside of the body in blood or any
other suitable soil it elongates into long undivided
chains, or threads in which brilliant spores appear
which are at last set free by the disintegration of the
bacillary filament. The oval spores, when placed in
proper soil, elongate at one end and change into growing rods which then pass through the same vital cycle.
The formation of spores is completed within about
twenty-four hours at the temperature of the animal
body. Cold retards this process and below 18° C.
sporification is no longer possible. The other limit of
temperature beyond which the production of seeds is
checked is about 42° to 44° C., varying with the
nature of the cultivating medium.

The bacillus anthracis is easily destroyed. Desicca-

*Deutche Med. Wodenschrift, 1881, p. 89.

tion kills it in a few days (or at the latest in a few
weeks in larger masses not quite dry in the interior).
A heat of 50° C. suffices for its destruction in twenty
minutes. Want of oxygen is fatal to it in some hours.
On the other hand the presence of oxygen in the
form of ozone is harmless.* But while the developed
form of this parasite is so easily killed, the spores
offer a great resistance to damaging influences. They
withstand permanent desiccation, or even alternate
moistening and drying, deprivation of oxygen, likewise any temperature below the boiling point (unless
the exposure is very long). Time seems to have no
effect upon their germinating power. No other pathogenic micro-organism can be as readily cultivated outside of the body as the bacillus anthracis. Almost
any animal juice, blood, broth, urine or aqueous humor
will suffice as a soil, if only neutral or slightly alkaline, likewise the infusion of many vegetables and
grasses.

These researches into the biology of the parasite,
mainly the work of Koch,† have established clearly
how the disease spreads. Apart from the intentional
inoculation the disease can be communicated by contact of any of the animal tissues or fluids which
contain the bacilli, with wounds. As Davaine has
shown the sting of wasps and other insects can transfer the virus from one animal to another. Man is not
infrequently infected by handling animal material, like
leather or wool, coming from diseased animals. In
many cases such material is so old and dry, that it
can no longer contain any living bacilli, but only
spores. Probably the infection by means of the de-

*Szpilman, Zeitschrift f. phys. Chemie. Bd. IV., p. 350.
†Cohn's Beitraege z. Biologie d. Pflanzen, Bd. II., Heft II., p. 177,
and Mittheil. aus d. k. Gesundheitsamte, p. 49.

veloped bacilli is a rare occurrence at the best on
account of their destructibility. But where the diseased animal dies, the discharges from the nose, mouth,
bladder and wounds all containing bacilli, impregnate
the soil. If the temperature is only above 18° C.
these bacilli soon develop spores, which then remain
in the field almost indestructible and can infect any
animals grazing there. Pasteur, who evidently overlooked the importance of the discharges deposited on
the surface of the soil, attributed an important role
to earth worms in transporting the spores from the
buried cadavers to the surface. But Koch has since
shown that this ingenious hypothesis is unnecessary.
For at the depth at which animal cadavers are usually
buried, viz.: half a metre or more below the surface,
the temperature in most European countries does not
rise above 18° C., and hence sporification would be
impossible in the cadaver. Moreover, the want of
oxygen would prevent the formation of spores at such
a depth, and does indeed kill the developed bacilli
within a short time. Hence we need not look for the
contagion below the surface of the earth.

Experience has shown, that the weather and the
nature of the soil exert an unmistakable influence on
the prevalence of anthrax. Warmth and moisture favor
its occurrence, while those farms are most dreaded as
"splenic-fever districts" which have an alkaline or
calcareous subsoil and are either marshy or subject to
occasional inundations. In some such localities the
disease persists as a frequent epidemic, although
cadavers of diseased animals may never have been
buried there. The explanation of these climatic and
telluric influences is evident, since Koch has shown
that the bacillus anthracis can vegetate outside of the
body of animals under conditions actually occurring in

nature. In the terminology of modern pathologists
the virus of this disease is both endogenous and ectogenous. It can vegetate and multiply in the body of
the victim, but it can also grow and increase outside
of it. The bacillus anthracis will readily develop in
many vegetable infusions. Such nutritive fluids it
finds in swamps and in pools of stagnant water, in
which dead plants are macerating, especially when the
vegetable acids are neutralized by the alkaline constituents of the soil. At any temperature above 18° C.
spores are formed, and when these almost indestructible seeds have once been distributed (for instance by
flooding) throughout a field, the germs of the disease
cannot be removed again from the locality by any
means yet known. The secret of the persistence of
the disease is the fact that the bacillus anthracis is
not limited to a parasitic mode of life in the animal
body, but can vegetate on the proper refuse, even
where no animals exist. It is a plant indigenous to
the soil of certain localities, passing but occasionally
and accidentally into the body of animals. There is
no evidence that the parasite is ever carried by the
air into the animal system.

The disease can be transferred to most animals
commonly used for experimentation. Rodents are
especially susceptible to it. Cats and dogs on the
other hand often resist an inoculation, especially when
not too young. According to Toussaint old dogs can
be infected with certainty only by intravenous injection.
Amongst the sheep, commonly the readiest victims of
this disease, Chauveau found a certain species imported
from Algiers, possessing an almost perfect immunity
against it. The pig also seems to be unable to contract it. In man the inoculation through a wound
produces at first only a local symptom—the malignant

pustule—from which he may recover without constitutional disease, on excision of the pustule or sometimes even spontaneously. Birds are not very liable to develop the disease on inoculation, though Oemler affirms that he has *often* succeeded in a variable percentage in chickens and other species. Pasteur on the other hand claims that under ordinary circumstances the fowl cannot be inoculated, for the high temperature of its body—42° C—is not favorable to the development of the parasite. But on cooling the body of the fowl by immersing the legs in cold water, he could infect it successfully and could thus let the disease run its fatal course, or could enable the chicken to recover by allowing it to regain its normal temperature in time. The great importance of this experimental result is evident. It appears very suggestive as to the direction in which therapeutic endeavors should be made in parasitic diseases. But unfortunately Pasteur* does not communicate the details of his experiments, and does not even state how often he has made this observation. Hence Koch denies its accuracy, both because Oemler could inoculate normal fowls (though not every time) and because the bacillus anthracis can yet grow at 42° C. Still Koch has not disproven Pasteur's claims by any personal research.

Gibier† has lately claimed that charbon can also be communicated to frogs (at least in some instances), but only when these animals are kept at a temperature of 35° to 37° C.

The bacillus anthracis can enter the system of a susceptible animal through almost any channel except the unbroken skin. As Buchner has shown even the

---

*Comptes Rendus, 1878, No. 2.
†Comptes Rendus, 1882, vol. 94, p. 1605.

inhalation of dried bacilli is fatal to mice, though
ordinarily this is not the mode of entrance of the
parasite. The natural infection occurs almost wholly
from the digestive tube, with the exception of occasional wounds and stings of insects. Toussaint*
claims, that the lymphatic glands in the infected
region indicate the point of entrance of the virus by
their swelling. By means of this guide he has traced
the origin of natural charbon to infection from the
mouth in some twelve sheep and a couple of cows.
Koch, however, in his latest work† disputes that the
mouth is the usual starting point of the disease, but
insists that in most instances the spores pass into the
small intestines and there germinate in the alkaline
contents, whereupon the bacilli penetrate through the
intestinal wall. At any rate, this is the mode of
infection in the so-called intestinal mycosis of man,
cases which cannot be diagnosed during life but
which the *post-mortem* reveals as genuine anthrax.

Like all infectious diseases, anthrax has a period of
incubation. This varies in length with the size of the
animal, as the theory of the nature of the disease
clearly indicates. For in order to produce a disturbance the number of bacilli in the system must bear
some proportion to the size of the invaded organism
and the multiplication of the parasites is, of course, a
question of time. Hence, while some twelve to eighteen hours elapse, before visible symptoms occur in the
rabbit, the stage of incubation requires some two or
three days in the case of a sheep. Moreover, this
latent period depends on the number of the parasites
introduced. The larger the quantity of virus injected,
the quicker is the fatal number of parasites obtained.

---

*Recherches experiment. sur la maladie charbonneuse, 1879.
†Ueber die Milzbrandimpfung, 1882.

The intravenous injection of the blood of an animal afflicted with the disease reproduces characteristic anthrax within some four or six hours, while on the other hand the inoculation of a few bacilli only prolongs the period of incubation by one or more days. This accounts for the protracted course of the natural infection as compared with the quicker death from experimental inoculation. For in the natural infection of anthrax and other diseases the number of parasites entering the system is probably quite small.

From the point of infection the bacilli pass to the nearest lymphatic glands, which by their swelling indicate the irritation caused by the growing parasites. It is only toward the end of the period of incubation, that the bacilli enter the blood in any appreciable number, and it is only some hours before death that the blood contains any large quantity of them. Moreover, this varies in different animals. In mice there may be very few or even none in the circulating blood even at the moment of death, which accounts for some of the older incorrect statements regarding the occurrence of splenic fever without the presence of the bacilli. The parasites are evidently arrested in the capillaries of most of the viscera, especially the spleen, where they continue their growth until they choke up these vessels completely. By appropriate staining Koch has shown that the "natural" injection by means of these bacilli demonstrates the topography of the capillaries more elegantly, than any artificial injection. Toussaint has watched the growth of the parasites in the living omentum spread out under the microscope. Wherever an extravasation occurs the bacilli pass into the surrounding tissues. It is probably thus that they get into the secretions, which are all tinged with blood. In the case of pregnant animals the placenta offers a barrier to the passage of the bacilli into the fœtal blood, hence, as Davaine and others have shown, the fœtus is as a rule not infected. But Strauss and Chamberland* have recently found that this is not invariably so, and that sometimes a few bacilli can be found in the fœtal blood (of guinea pigs).

It is not yet settled in what manner the growth of the parasite destroys the host's life. The dark color of the blood even during life has led Pasteur and others to suppose that the parasites, which are known to have a strong affinity for oxygen, abstract this gas from the blood and thereby asphyxiate the animal in a slow manner. Still this view has not been proven experimentally. At any rate, the growth of so large a mass of parasites in the living blood-vessels cannot but injure the animal organism, be it by the abstraction of oxygen or nourishment, by the embolism of so many capillaries or by the formation of bacterial products poisonous to the victim.

Anthrax is usually a fatal disease, at least in the herbivora. But, if the victim does recover it is not liable to contract the disease again. The first attack gives immunity against a return of the disease, at any rate in cattle and sheep. But this immunity does not occur in all animal species. Loeffler† quotes Oemler in proof of the possibility of repeated attacks of malignant pustule in man. In his own experiments he found that rats, which are not very susceptible animals, can be inoculated a number of times with either slight or no effect at all, and will still succumb at some later occasion. According to Koch‡ similar experiments (with mitigated virus) have since been made at the

---

*Comptes Rendus, Vol. 95, p. 1290.
†Mittheil. aus. d. k. Gesundheitsamte, p. 156.
‡Ueber d. Milzbrandimpfung.

laboratory of the German board of health on rabbits, guinea pigs and mice, showing that these animals also cannot acquire a perfect immunity.

The immunity which cattle and sheep obtain by a first non-fatal attack of charbon suggested researches in the hope of producing the disease in a modified form. For Pasteur had just then shown that in another infectious disease — chicken-cholera — the virus can be so mitigated as to cause only a mild attack, which secures immunity against a subsequent return of the disease. In short he had proven the possibility of transforming a disastrous virus into a comparatively harmless "vaccine" matter. Toussaint was the first to attempt this in the case of anthrax. He heated blood of anthrax to 55° C. for ten minutes or filtered it through several layers of filter paper, or added one per cent. of carbolic acid and claimed to reduce thereby its virulence, so that an injection of it gave rise only to a slight disturbance, followed by immunity against the disease. But a repetition of his experiments by Loeffler proved them to be unreliable, if not fallacious, which is also the criticism of Pasteur on them. Pasteur himself soon afterwards devised a method by which the desired result could be accomplished.* In the case of the chicken-cholera parasite Pasteur had reduced its virulence to animals by prolonged exposure to the air without change of soil. This procedure could not be utilized in the case of the bacillus anthracis on account of the speedy transition of the latter into the state of dormant vitality, viz.: by the formation of spores. But sporification is prevented by a temperature which by itself does not kill the bacilli. Kept permanently at a temperature

---

*Various communications to the Paris Academy of Sciences, 1881 and 1882.

of 42°–43° C. in neutralized chicken-broth, this bacillus does not produce spores according to Pasteur. Under these circumstances its vitality is gradually lowered and within a period of one month it dies. Inoculated in animals during any time before its ultimate death the bacillus will still cause anthrax, but with a severity proportionate to the vitality of the micro-organism. The disease can thus be obtained in any desired degree of intensity. The feeble attack of charbon from which the animal recovers, confers upon it an immunity somewhat proportionate to the severity of the experimental disease. The immunity granted by a single attack of the milder type is not absolute, however. But it can be made so by a subsequent inoculation with a more active virus. Pasteur soon extended his experiments to entire flocks of animals and proved on a large scale that cattle and sheep, which have been "vaccinated" twice at intervals of twelve days with the attenuated bacillus anthracis can now resist successfully an inoculation with the most active anthrax material. He has cultivated the parasite in the above described manner on a large scale and puts into the market a "first vaccine" as the result of twenty-four days' attenuation, while the "second vaccine" is only enfeebled by a cultivation of twelve days at a high temperature. The power of reproduction of the enfeebled parasite is not materially lessened, nor are its appearances altered. Like the original bacillus anthracis it produces spores at a suitable temperature, but these spores and the fresh crop of bacilli developed from them have only the virulence of the enfeebled virus. Their power of struggling with the animal cells has been permanently diminished in proportion to the length .of time, during which they had been cultivated under circumstances

unfavorable to them. The inoculation is performed by
injecting under the skin a few grams of the chicken-
broth containing the mitigated bacilli. The disturbance which they produce in the animal is simply a
more or less severe fever. These discoveries have
opened up an entirely new prospect in the manage-
ment of infectious diseases and their importance is
simply fundamental.

Pasteur has published numerous statistics of the
wholesale employment of this protective vaccination.
His most recent report refers to the results obtained
in the department d'Eure et Loire.* Altogether 79,392
sheep were vaccinated, amongst which number the
loss by splenic fever was reduced to 0.65 per cent.
in the course of the past year. In former years the
average loss had been 9.01 per cent., though during
the past year the dampness of the season would probably have given rise only to some 3 per cent. of loss,
as calculated on the basis of former experience. Indeed, in those herds in which only a part of
the animals were protected by vaccination the loss
amongst 1,659 unprotected sheep was only 3.9 per
cent. while of 2,308 vaccinated animals but eight
(0.4 per cent.) died of anthrax. Four thousand five
hundred and sixty-two cattle had also been vaccinated,
of which but 0.24 per cent. succumbed to the disease,
while former years had given a loss of 7.03 per cent.

Very serious objections, however, have been urged
by Koch† against the practical application of Pasteur's researches. He does not underrate their great
theoretical value, but denies that they are complete
enough for immediate practical utilization. He points
out, first of all, that in other animals but cattle and

*Comptes Rendus. Vol. 95, p. 1250.
†Ueber die Milzbrandimpfung.

sheep even the severest non-fatal attack of anthrax
does not confer immunity. The "attenuated virus"
which Pasteur puts into the market for the vaccination of herds, Koch claims is not always of the
proper strength; sometimes it is so feeble as to fail
in its purpose of protecting the animals, while in
other instances it was virulent enough to produce up to
10 or even 15 per cent. of loss by the vaccination itself.
In his repetition of Pasteur's experiments he found that
virus most suitable for the first vaccination of sheep,
which still killed mice on inoculation, but failed to
give anthrax to guinea-pigs. The second vaccination
is just severe enough to grant immunity against
further inoculation, and not intense enough to kill
the sheep, if the bacilli are only enfeebled to such
an extent as not to infect the rabbit, but can still
vegetate in and destroy the guinea-pig. But the
most fatal objection which Koch raises is the statement that the immunity produced by the protective
vaccination refers only to the inoculation through
wounds and *not to the natural infection with anthrax
through the intestinal canal.* If this be really so—
and both the observations in France, at Kapuvar
(Hungary) and at Packisch (Saxony), as well as
Koch's experiments prove that the immunity is at
least not absolute—then the practical value of
Pasteur's vaccinations is as yet chimerical. Koch
tested the immunity of eight sheep vaccinated twice
according to Pasteur's directions by inoculating them
with material from an animal just dead of anthrax.
One of the victims died, the other seven resisted
successfully, and had thus passed through three
vaccinations. Twelve days later they were *fed* with
spores cultivated from the material used for the last
inoculation, in consequence of which two succumbed

to the infection. The "natural" mode of infection is therefore the most dangerous to the animal and cannot be absolutely prevented by protective vaccination. That a difference does exist between infection from a wound and the entrance of the parasite through the alimentary canal, is evident indeed from various experiments on cattle, animals most prone to the natural infection. In the different inoculations made by Pasteur on French farms, and by his assistant in Kapuvar (Hungary), very few of the non-protected cattle died from the effects of the virulent anthrax material, and not even all took sick. Similar observations have also been made by Chauveau,* and yet all cattle-raisers dread the so-frequent natural infection.

It is likely that the virulence of the bacillus anthracis, its power to struggle successfully with the animal cells, can be reduced in different manners. Pasteur's assertion that it is the influence of the oxygen in his mode of cultivation, which enfeebles its vitality is not really supported by any proofs. Koch attributes the "attenuation" rather to the high temperature, for the length of time necessary to deprive the bacillus of its virulence varies in inverse proportion to the temperature at which it is kept. Toussaint's original claim that the anthrax virus could be reduced to a "vaccine" by heating it to 55° C., it is true, was not confirmed by the Berlin experimenters, but they made use only of rodents and not the animals—sheep—which Toussaint himself employed. Chauveau† has since repeated the experiments on sheep, and finds them correct, if but both the temperature and the time of exposure be taken into

*Comptes Rendus, 1880, Vol. 90, p. 648.
†Comptes Rendus, 1882, Vol. 94, p. 1694.

7

account. By enclosing the blood containing the bacilli in very thin closed glass pipettes and immersing them entirely in the water-bath, he found that even 50° C. sufficed to kill the parasite if the exposure lasted twenty minutes. During this period its virulence diminishes gradually, so that when inoculated it produces a modified form of anthrax, of a severity inversely proportionate to the length of time it was heated. The disease modified by this mode of precedure was found to be equally efficient as a protection against subsequent attacks as that produced by Pasteur's method—at least as far as the experimental inoculation under the skin was concerned. A difference between Pasteur's and Chauveau's observations is the fact, that the bacilli heated to 50° C. do not multiply as rapidly, when subsequently kept at a suitable temperature as they did prior to this exposure. Their power of reproduction is enfeebled like their virulence. In what manner the influence of heat or other damaging agencies can reduce the virulence of the parasite has not yet been solved. As long as we are ignorant of the nature of the attack and the defense in the struggle between parasites and animal tissues neither the above question, nor the query, as to the essence of the immunity against a return of the disease can be answered.

In this connection I must refer briefly to some researches by Buchner.* His object was not merely to modify the properties of the bacillus anthracis, but to prove its identity with the common hay bacillus, an organism harmless to animals. He wished to demonstrate the truth of Naegeli's view, that one bacterial variety can be converted into another by adaptation to the conditions of nutrition. For this purpose the

*Sitzungsberichte der Muenchener Akademie, 1880. Heft III.

bacillus anthracis was cultivated in a solution of meat
extract and transferred into a fresh soil from day to
day, while oxygen was freely supplied by shaking
the vessel. In the course of thirty-six generations its
virulence was so reduced, that it required very large
quantities of the fluid to produce anthrax in mice.
The cultivation during about half a year deprived it
entirely of the power of vegetating in the animal
body. Conversely the genuine hay bacilli were grown
in fresh rabbit's blood after adaptation to an alkaline
soil by cultivation in egg albumen. Nourished in this
manner they ultimately acquired virulence and produced in mice a disease like anthrax. But these
results have been severely criticized by Koch.* Since
Buchner did not use staining methods he could not
prove at all the identity or non-identity of one or the
other species. For minor differences in form cannot
be recognized in the fresh specimen. Koch claims
further, that there is no positive proof that the micro-
organisms met with ultimately in either series of experiments were the result of a transformation, while
there is reason to believe that they got there by substitution. In view of the importance of these results
—if true—Koch demands absolute security against the
accidental admission of other germs, which guarantee
Buchner has not given. In Koch's experiments the
bacillus anthracis was cultivated in one hundred and
fifteen successive generations on a solid soil (potato-
slice) without losing its virulence to any extent. Koch
points out also that the virulent bacillus supposed to
have resulted from a gradual transformation of the
hay bacillus, may not have been the bacillus anthracis,
but another parasite the germs of which are very
freely disseminated throughout nature. The disease

---

*Mittheilungen, etc., p. 68.

this produces — malignant œdema — cannot be distinguished from anthrax in mice, although there is quite a difference in larger animals.　These remarks of Koch's apply equally to the experiments of Koehler,* who also claimed, that he had transformed the bacillus. subtilis into a virulent parasite by continued cultivation in blood.

Buchner, however, has since published new researches† corroborative of his former results.　But even in these I can detect a serious flaw, viz.: the use of non-sterilized fluids.　The bacillus anthracis was sown in solutions of meat-extract containing an addition of finely subdivided yolk of egg with some free alkali.　By cultivation in this fluid continued for a few days it changed in appearance and properties.　It lost its virulence to animals, it grew no longer in the form of flakes at the bottom of the fluid, but was diffused throughout the solution or even formed a scum on the surface like the true hay bacillus.　Moreover, it acquired a distinct though sluggish mobility.　In short, Buchner claims that he can thus transform the anthrax parasite through a series of intervening steps into the hay bacillus.　Though these later experiments appear more precise than his former ones, they still lack the necessary stamp of scientific accuracy to be accepted without further confirmation.

An affection the nature of which has been as well investigated as that of anthrax ought to be a "test disease" for therapeutic action.　But unfortunately nothing can be done as yet for the cure of this disease.　When it remains localized at first, as in man, a sufficiently early excision of the pustule stops the progress, though a spontaneous recovery may also

---

*Der Heupilz, etc.　Inaug. Diss. Gœttingen, 1881.
†Sitzungsberichte der Muenchener Akademie, 1882.　Heft. II.

occur, but when the bacilli have once invaded the blood-vessels, we can do nothing more to aid the animal tissues in their struggle. Having learned the remarkable antiseptic properties of corrosive sublimate, Koch has tried its use in experimental anthrax. Since it interferes with the growth of the parasite when present to the extent of one part in 600,000, and arrests the development completely in the strength of one part in 330,000, a sufficient quantity can be injected into animals to demonstrate its antiseptic property without killing them. But the introduction of 0.5 to 1 milligram of corrosive sublimate under the skin of guinea pigs weighing 600 to 700 grams influenced neither the previous nor the subsequent inoculation with the bacillus anthracis. Probably the mercurial salt enters into new combinations with the animal fluids, which are not equally destructive to the parasite.

CHICKEN CHOLERA

is a second instance of a disease traced to the invasion of the body by bacteria in a manner beyond dispute. It is an affection peculiar to fowl, though transferable to other birds and even to some mammals. The most striking symptom is somnolence, which augments up to the death of the animal occurring in from one to three days. The autopsy shows as the most striking lesion a violent inflammation of the intestines. In this disease micro-organisms had been seen by Moritz, Perroncito and by Toussaint, but their significance has been mainly proven by Pasteur* by cultivation, isolation and inoculation of the parasites. He describes them as small "vibrios"

---

*In several communications to the Paris Academy of Sciences in 1880 and 1881.

of the shape of a figure 8, in other words diplococci, but gives no further details of their appearance. They abound in the blood and tissues of the diseased fowl. They are contained in the evacuations of the animal and pass thus from one to another, entering through the alimentary canal.' Artificial inoculation, however, can be made through any wound.

The parasites grow readily in neutralized (and sterilized) chicken-broth, but not at all in simpler solutions like urine or yeast decoction. In fact Pasteur uses the latter fluid, known as a good soil for many bacteria, as a test for the purity of his culture. For while the disease-germs do not grow in it, any accidental bacterial "impurities" will readily develop there. Chicken-broth is rendered turbid in some hours by the cholera bacteria, but the growth ceases about the fourth day (at the proper temperature), whereupon the parasites settle to the bottom in the form of minute separate micrococci. Pasteur has traced this limitation of development to exhaustion of the soil, and not to the excretion of products injurious to the parasites. For when he filtered them off through a layer of plaster of paris, and thereupon evaporated the chicken-broth at a low temperature in the vacuum, the re-solution of this residue in a fresh solution did not render the fluid unfit as a soil for another crop. Pasteur tested also the effect upon animals of the fluid in which the bacteria had grown, but from which they had been removed by filtration. He found that the injection of this fluid *in the proper quantity* could produce the principal symptom of the disease, viz.: somnolence, from which, however, the chicken recovered in some hours. But this was not the disease, not an infection, simply a temporary poisoning by one of the bacterial products. Evidently the parasites secrete certain substances, both in the animal body and in the cultivating flask, which exert a soporific effect upon fowls. The blood of the animal thus poisoned, contains no micrococci and is not infectious.

Inoculation, however, of the cultivated parasite reproduced the disease in all its virulence, no matter how often it had been transplanted from one flask to another. In guinea-pigs the inoculation provoked only a localized abscess without further impairment of the animal's health, but the pus of this abscess contained the parasite in its unaltered virulence to fowls. In the rabbit, however, a constitutional fatal disease is produced, which Toussaint* claims is but a form of septicæmia. Though Pasteur denies this, it seems to me but a quibble about words, as long as neither affection is absolutely characterized by any local lesion.

The special interest in chicken cholera centers in Pasteur's discovery how to modify and mitigate the virulence of the parasites. It was the first experimental proof, that "the virus" of a disease can be altered in strength. Pasteur observed, that while the parasite retained all its properties, when kept in the state of vegetation by frequent change of soil, its prolonged sojourn in an exhausted soil enfeebled it. When the exhaustion of the chicken-broth prevented it from growing any longer, its vitality began to fail in proportion to the length of time. When generation succeeds generation the influence of time is not felt, but when the growth ceases the micro-organism ages. In the course of some nine months it dies. Pasteur attributed this reduction of vitality to the influence of the atmospheric oxygen. For when he sealed his

*Comptes Rendus, 1881, Vol. 93, p. 219.

vessels hermetically, time seemed to exert no influence upon the vitality of these parasites.

The inoculation of fowls with the ageing parasite produces a modified disease, the severity of which diminishes with the time the micro-organism has been kept in an unchanged soil. The attack becomes less fatal to the animals and in its milder form amounts simply to a localized necrosis of the muscle where the inoculation is made. A muscular sequestrum is formed, which is removed by slight suppuration. In the mildest form produced by means of the most "attenuated" virus even the local lesion is but very slight, and the animal always recovers. After the parasite has once attained a certain degree of attenuation, it can be kept at that standard of virulence by further cultivation in a fresh soil, if only transferred to a new flask as soon as it has exhausted the first solution. If allowed to remain again in one and the same fluid without change, its vitality is further reduced. On the other hand Pasteur could again augment its virulence by cultivating it in the body of animals, which it is yet capable of destroying. When the virus has ceased to be fatal to fowls it can still kill the more susceptible sparrow, especially when but a few days of age. By thus passing the parasite through the body of a young sparrow to an old sparrow and thence to a chicken it regains again sufficient virulence to struggle successfully with the fowl's tissues.

A chicken which has recovered from an attack of cholera is no longer susceptible to the disease. The parasite, which has once been overcome by the animal's body cannot gain a foothold a second time, though a more virulent virus may yet affect the animals. In other words the immunity granted by a mild attack of the disease is not absolute. But it can be made so by repeated vaccination. Pasteur claims, indeed, that the immunity can be acquired by the animal without any suffering. For by choosing the most attenuated parasite for the first inoculation the animal is scarcely affected. Though it would yet succumb to the introduction of the most powerful virus, it can, however, withstand without danger a second vaccination with a·medium grade of parasites. This second, or at the most a third inoculation with more virulent material gives it thenceforth absolute immunity against the disease without any of the attacks having been severe.

I have not been able to learn whether Pasteur's vaccinations have yet been practiced on any extensive scale for combatting this scourge of the barnyards. But he has also indicated another plan of exterminating the disease which seems more economical. The parasite is conveyed from chicken to chicken mainly in the excretions which become mingled with the food. The micrococcus can be readily killed by dilute acids, one part of sulphuric acid in a thousand of water being sufficient for this purpose. Hence by removing the infected and diseased animals and flooding the grounds with such acidulated water the source of infection is taken away.

· LECTURE V.

Surgical Infections. — Aseptic Wounds. — Suppuration. — Abscesses.—
Furuncles. — Osteomyelitis. — Pyæmia. — Decomposition of Pus.
—Traumatic Fever. — Putrid Poisoning. — Septicæmia.

SURGICAL INFECTIONS.

Under this, heading it may be convenient to group
together a number of disorders, which may occur as
complications of open wounds. This classification is
of course an arbitrary one. For the only common
bond of union in the nature of these diseases is the
fact, that they are due to germs, which usually, enter
the body through wounds. The scarcity of these
affections in certain localities and their prevalence in
others when once started there, suggested the view to
former surgeons, that they took their start in something in the air entering the wounds. Indeed this
explanation forces itself upon the observer on reflect-
ing upon the invariable benignant course of wounds
not in communication with the air, *i. e.*, fractures of
bones and ruptures of soft parts without destruction
of the continuity of the skin. This observation
naturally led to the introduction of subcutaneous

surgery, which, wherever applicable, produces wounds, that heal as kindly as those not extending to the surface of the body. But the credit of having clearly recognized that the "something" in the air so dangerous to wounds, are living beings, bacteria or their germs, and that it must be the aim of the surgeon to exclude these from the wound, belongs to Joseph Lister. Just prior to his own studies on wounds, Pasteur had demonstrated in the most conclusive manner, that all putrefaction is due to micro-organisms, and that the germs of these beings are disseminated throughout the air. It is an evident surgical observation that the occurrence of putrefactive processes in wounds retards their healing. It had been shown, moreover, by numerous experimenters, that the injection of putrid substances into the bodies of animals produces disorders resembling the complications of wounds most dreaded by the surgeon, viz: progressive inflammations and septicæmia. Starting from these premises, Lister began experimenting with various forms of dressings for wounds, with the intention of keeping out the germs of the air, and to destroy them if they had gained access. For this purpose antiseptic substances—principally carbolic acid —were employed. Lister does not claim to have been the first to employ carbolic acid in wounds, but in spite of all attempts to belittle his methods he *was the first to use carbolic acid with the distinct aim of making the dressing a barrier to the entrance of germs.* His methods were not born complete, but were more and more perfected in the course of painstaking observations. Lister does not seem to have made many microscopic observations of wounds with reference to the presence of germs, he acted rather with a happy intuition on the basis of the results of his predecessors. His own practical results, however, have more than justified his anticipations. They have brought us to the threshold of a new era in surgery. The surgeon of yore did his best in the performance of the necessary operation, but the results following his wounds he could not control. The surgeon of to-day, however, is responsible for the course of the wound he inflicts. Any untoward accident starting from the wound is due to his want of care.

A wound which follows a truly aseptic course, *i. e.*, from which germs are wholly excluded, is not a source of danger to the organism, provided it does not destroy life directly, by involving some organ of vital importance. Such an aseptic wound is almost painless; its edges are not red, inflamed or swollen. If there is any discharge at all, it is only an oozing of clear fluid, for the very appearance of pus indicates, that it is not wholly aseptic. The wounded surfaces will invariably grow together, if they can be put in contact, while if a gap exists, this is filled up by granulations without any other disturbance of the wound. No constitutional disturbance is created by such a wound. If fever exists at all, it is very slight and not accompanied by any interference with the general health. The occurrence of such a mild fever without disturbance of the well-being of the patient— termed by Volkmann aseptic fever—is not indicative of the presence of germs in the wound. It is probably due to the absorption of extravasated blood.

This description of an ideal wound, is not a creation of the fancy; *it applies accurately to every wound successfully protected by a typical Lister dressing*, or some other thoroughly aseptic mode of treatment, for instance by the application of iodoform. Whenever a wound pains, is inflamed, secretes pus and produces

disturbance of the health, the dictates of antiseptic
surgery have not been carried out. It is not the loss
of continuity which causes the local disturbance or
the constitutional disease, but it is the vegetation of
bacteria in the wound which proves so disastrous.
The truly aseptic wound, even if of considerable
magnitude does not annoy the patient as much as
does a scratch on your finger, unheeded by most of
you, yet appealing to your attention by reason of the
uncomfortable itching, and the tenderness—slight
though it be—in its vicinity. The faint redness of
the edges of such a scratch indicates that the surface
of this miniature wound is irritated by "something."
Although I do not know of any direct observations, I
have no doubt that this "something" is the vegetation of bacteria in, and under the scab. For Koch
found, that even the track of the hypodermic needle
remains visible in the tissues, by reason of the
growth of bacteria along this capillary channel.*

The presence of bacteria is never quite indifferent
as far as the healing of a wound is concerned. Yet
since there are different species of bacteria the amount
and nature of the disturbance depends upon the
variety present. Cheyne† found a micrococcus, the
dimensions of which he does not detail, occasionally
in wounds which apparently followed an aseptic course.
Its presence may be indicated by a sour smell, but it
does not seem to irritate the wound perceptibly. Micro-organisms had also been found formerly in some
aseptic wounds by Ranke and by Schueller, but the
results of these observers are less accurate, since
they did not use any staining methods in order to
determine the form of the bacteria. Moreover, doubts

*Mittheilungen a. d. k. Gesundheitsamte, p. 118.
†Antiseptic Surgery, chap. XII.

are permissible, whether these authors dealt with completely aseptic wounds at a time, when antiseptic surgery was a comparatively new · feature in Germany.
But according to the observations of Cheyne on Lister's patients the majority of aseptic wounds harbor no
bacteria whatever.

When suppuration occurs it is always due to some
irritation of the wound. But it cannot be said that
pus is produced only through the action of bacteria.
It is, on the contrary, quite likely that the presence of
any chemical substance sufficiently irritating leads to
suppuration. · Recently Uskoff* has attempted to learn
whether suppuration is invariably accompanied by bacteria. In order to decide this point injections of
different fluids were made under the skin of animals,
and if any suppuration followed, the pus and sections
from the inflamed tissues were examined microscopically with Koch's mode of illumination after staining.
Fluids innocuous by themselves, like water or milk,
produced abscesses only when injected repeatedly in
large quantities. In such pus micrococci were invariably found. The fluids had been heated, but the
author himself doubts his success in sterilizing them.
Possibly the bacteria entered through the wound
made by the needle. Orthman† has just published a
repetition of these experiments, in which he learned that
the injection of non-irritating fluids—if performed with
strict aseptic precautions—never causes abscesses, no
matter how large the quantity. But when irritating
substances like turpentine or croton oil were applied,
the abscesses which followed did not contain any bacteria, nor were these found in the surrounding tissues.
Hence it is proven, that suppuration follows any suf-

*Virchow's Archiv. f. path. Anatomie, Vol. 86, p. 150.
†Virchow's Archiv, Bd. 90., p. 549.

ficient irritation of the tissues, be it by the growth of certain bacteria, or by the presence of any irritant chemical substance.

It is quite questionable whether mechanical irritation alone suffices to produce suppuration. At any rate it is well known, that foreign bodies can remain within the tissues without causing purulent inflammation, provided only they contain no germs. Suppuration is likewise not the inevitable consequence of the presence of a dead tissue in the interior of the body. Thus obliteration of the artery of the testicle, or of the kidney, causes death of these organs, but if bacteria be excluded the dead tissue is gradually absorbed without suppuration. Occasionally the flaps of an aseptic amputation wound mortify from insufficient blood supply, but no further disturbance is caused by this accident if the antiseptic dressing fulfills its purpose. It has likewise been learned in various recent pathological studies, that bits of tissue hardened in alcohol can be put under the skin, or into the peritoneal cavity, with antiseptic precautions, and are absorbed there without producing inflammation.

SUPPURATION

can be caused, however, by the presence of certain bacteria in the tissues, as has been definitely demonstrated by Ogston.* In 100 instances of acute abscesses, previously unopened, this observer never failed to find micrococci in the pus. These organisms, of various sizes, from $\frac{1}{750}$ to $\frac{1}{1480}$ of a millimeter, were united either in chains or in groups. The mode of grouping seemed to indicate a difference in the species, for it was reproduced on cultivating the micrococcus either

*British Medical Journal, March 12th, 1881.

in or outside of the body. But no difference could be detected between the action of the chain or the cluster form. The number of microccoci present in the pus varied immensely in different instances. Ogston gives the extremes as 900 to 45,000,000 of micrococci per cubic millimeter of pus, though his counting method does not deserve much confidence. The microccoci were mostly found in the fluid, but sometimes in the pus cells. They possessed an apparently active vital movement. In stained sections of the tissues around the abscess, coccus-infiltration was observed. In the pus coming from catarrhal mucus membranes the same organisms were found. They were likewise never absent in the pus of ulcers and suppurating wounds (96 observations), and indeed their number was proportionate to the intensity of the suppuration. Whenever a wound smelled suspiciously other bacteria were also present in large numbers. In thirteen chronic abscesses, however, no micro-organisms were found by means of the staining methods and Abbe's condensor. Whether they had been there originally the author does not try to decide.

The injection of the pus from the chronic abscesses proved harmless to animals. It was absorbed without reaction. Similarly innocuous was the injection of pus, the microccoci of which had been killed by the addition of an equal quantity of a 5 per cent. solution of carbolic acid, or by exposure to 55°C. Pus, however, of acute abscesses, containing living micrococci, invariably produced disastrous consequences, when injected under the skin of guinea-pigs and mice. It was only when less than $\frac{1}{16}$ of a minim was employed, that no reaction followed. Any larger quantity produced symptoms of blood-poisoning. The animals refused food, cowered down and were listless, but usu-

ally recovered after the lapse of from five to seven days.
The blood contained numerous micrococci during their
illness, but not after their recovery. The spot, where
the pus had been injected became red and swollen,
and within a few days an abscess was formed, in the
pus of which the micrococci existed in large numbers.
These parasites were also seen growing in the midst
of the surrounding tissues, upon which they seemed
to exert a destructive influence, for the tissues were
more waxy in aspect than normally. But by the
time the growth of the abscess was checked and it
became surrounded by a wall of granulation tissue,
this seemed to act as a barrier to the further invasion
of the tissues by the micrococci. On the inner surface of the abscess-wall they formed a thin, not continuous, layer.

Ogston's attempts to cultivate these micrococci outside the body were at first unsuccessful. Although he
used as soil a variety of fluids the micro-organisms did
not grow at all—or at least not actively—in any of
them. He attributes this to the fact that these beings
are anærobes—in the sense of Pasteur—and cannot
thrive in the presence of free oxygen. In confirmation of his view he states that the micrococci growing
on the surface of wounds exposed to the air, do
not produce inflammatory reaction with such certainty,
when injected under the skin, as does the pus of
closed abscesses. Cheyne has since doubted the correctness of this view, because he has sometimes succeeded in growing the micrococci from abscesses in
cucumber infusions. He is of the opinion, that they
did not grow in Ogston's experiments, because they
are often dead in the pus, when an abscess is opened.
But since Ogston states, that the micrococci possessed
active movements, this objection is not valid. Besides ·

Cheyne seems to have made use of thicker strata of fluid than Ogston, and the latter states that the micrococci do sometimes grow in the depth of the cultivating solution. Moreover Ogston did succeed in cultivating these bacteria away from the air in the interior of eggs, and the micrococci which had grown successively in two eggs were as virulent to animals as the original pus.

These researches establish definitely, that suppuration is almost always due to the growth of a certain micrococcus. It is easy to understand how this parasite can obtain access to wounds, especially when we consider, that its entrance into them can be prevented with certainty by the antiseptic precautions of Lister. Though the influence of the air may enfeeble the parasite in the pus on the surface, it cannot reach it in the interior of the tissues, which it invades. There its virulence can only be checked by the resistance of the living cells of the body. This resistance shows itself both in the limitation of the spreading of an abscess, and in the harmlessness of injections of minute quantities of pus. It is not so clear how the parasite gets into the system in order to produce an abscess. There is no evidence that it ordinarily reaches the locality where it grows, through the circulation. It is more likely that the micrococcus enters from some surface through a slight abrasion, for observant surgeons can frequently trace abscesses to such overlooked scratches.

It is not unlikely that other bacteria besides the micrococcus of Ogston may produce suppuration in certain cases. Thus Pasteur describes a different "vibrio" as the cause of suppuration. In a paper read at the French Academy of Medicine (April 30, 1878) he describes this bacterium as a short rod — in his words, sausage-like—at first freely moving, but at rest after growing for some time, slightly constricted in its centre and not unlike the common bacterium termo. Since Pasteur's description of the form of bacteria is never very close, it would be difficult to identify this micro-organism. He has met with it in the hydrant water of Paris, and cultivated it in meat infusion. It is said to be either aerobic or anærobic, according to the circumstances. When injected into the bodies of guinea-pigs it gave rise to abscesses the pus of which contained these micro-organisms. The inoculation with this pus started fresh abscesses. When large numbers of the parasite were used for inoculation portions of them were taken up by the circulation and deposited in other tissues, causing thus metastatic abscesses. Since the occurrence of multiple suppuration in different localities in consequence of infection from a primary seat of purulent inflammation characterizes *pyæmia*, Pasteur does not hesitate to consider this parasite as the cause of that disease. It is interesting to note that the injection of a *large* quantity of these bacteria is not harmless, even when their vitality has been destroyed by boiling. Their dead bodies are sufficiently irritant to provoke a suppurative inflammation, but such an abscess has no tendency to spread, and its pus is not infectious to other animals. Pasteur supposes, that the dead bacteria act as foreign bodies; but as foreign bodies are not irritant, if insoluble, it is more likely, that the living bacteria act upon the tissues by the secretion of some acrid substance, of which some remains in their dead bodies.

Pasteur has also found another micro-organism as the cause of suppuration, viz.: in *furuncles*. He figures it as a micrococcus in twos or fours, which he detected in the pus of unopened boils. His description applies

fully to the micrococcus found by Ogston in abscesses.
Yet it must be remembered that a furuncle differs
from an abscess to the extent of containing a necrosed
plug in its centre. Whether this is a peculiarity due
to the location of the furuncle in the skin or not, is
not yet decided. Pasteur* cultivated this micro-organism in chicken broth, or yeast infusion. When injected
into the bodies of rabbits and guinea-pigs it produced
abscesses. Its introduction, however, into the blood-
vessels proved harmless in these animals. The same
micro-organism was detected by Pasteur in the pus of
suppurative inflammation of the marrow-cavity of
bones, or

OSTEOMYELITIS.

It seems that he examined only one case of this
disease. In this instance the pus was literally an
emulsion of micrococci. A similar observation has been
made by Schueller.† The parasitic origin of osteomyelitis has also been claimed by Kocher‡ on the basis
of experiments. The injection of caustic substances
and irritants into the marrow of bones did not suffice
to produce osteomyelitis in dogs, as long as the injection was performed antiseptically. The only result was
a proliferation of the bone tissue obliterating the
cavity—technically termed sclerosis. But a true suppurative osteomyelitis could be brought on by the
injection of putrid solutions into the marrow, though
not in every instance. The material employed had
rotted in closed vessels without access of oxygen, and
contained mainly a long form of bacilli bearing spores
at their ends. Kocher was evidently of the opinion,

---

*Comptes Rendus de l' Academie d' Sciences. 1880. Vol. 90, p. 1033.
†Centralblatt f. Chirurgie, 1881, No. 42.
‡Archiv f. klin. Chirurgie.   Vol. 23, p. 101.

that the parasites producing osteomyelitis were identical with the agents of putrefaction. But he furnishes no proof for this view, as he does not give any description of the micro-organisms found in the pus. It is more in conformity with our present knowledge to suppose that the fluids employed, which were not pure cultures, contained some pathogenic germs. These were evidently few in number and not always present, for he did not get osteomyelitis in every instance of infection. Kocher calls attention to the fact that the disease—osteomyelitis—may vary very much in intensity and that it has a tendency to be complicated with secondary suppurations in other parts of the body. It is thus very difficult to draw a sharp line between complicated osteomyelitis and typical

PYÆMIA.

The clinical diagnosis of this latter form of blood-poisoning is beset with difficulties at the best. The only characteristic symptoms are the irregular fluctuations in the course of the fever, preceded usually by severe chills. But unless pyæmia begins with a distinct chill it is impossible to state the moment of its onset, and if the patient survives, the diagnosis is again involved in doubt. The disease is sharply characterized only by the post-mortem examination, which reveals secondary- or so-called metastatic—foci of suppuration in different internal organs, and suppurative inflammation of serous membranes.

The former view which gave the name to this disease, viz: that these metastatic suppurations are due to the entrance of pus into the veins from the original wound, has long been disproven by Virchow and others. Ordinary pus does not provoke pyæmia, when injected into the vessels. It requires the presence of a specific "something" in the pus to produce this result. This was most apparent in the experiments of Chauveau,* in which fresh, so-called healthy pus was injected into the carotid artery of horses and asses. The injection produced purulent inflammation in the organs directly reached by the pus, viz: the brain and eye, but the suppuration did not extend secondarily to other organs.

It has indeed long been known, that micro-organisms occur invariably in pyæmia. Reindfleisch stated in 1866, that the smaller metastatic deposits of the size of a pin's head, found especially in the substance of the heart in the form of softened yellow spots, consist entirely of "vibriones." He gives no further description of these parasites, even in the last edition of his "Pathological Anatomy." Subsequently both Von Recklinghausen and Waldeyer found colonies of micrococci in the blood-vessels and in the tissues in pyæmia. Micrococci have also been seen by Vogt in the blood of the living pyæmic patient, distributed irregularly throughout the fluid. In the wounds which gave rise to pyæmia bacteria were abundantly found by Birch–Hirschfeld, particularly in the form of micrococci in zoogloea masses. Similar observations had also been made by Klebs, who found bacterial masses adherent to the surface of the wound. He described both rod-shaped and globular organisms, and considering them genetically related to each other, termed them microsporon septicum. But he has never given satisfactory proof, that the various forms he described are really different stages of the same organism. He traced, however, the entrance of micrococci into the interspaces of the tissues surrounding the wounds, and into eroded veins. It is well known,

---

*Revue Scientifique, 1875.

that pyæmia often starts from a thrombosis of a vein next to the wound. In the clot of such veins Klebs and others have found micrococcus colonies, and the same micro-organisms are met with in the particles torn off from this clot by the blood current, and deposited in various parts of the system in the form of emboli. All these observations have been confirmed by other authors* and I do not know of any instances in which micro-organisms were not found in the pyæmic foci, when properly sought for. But I can find no description of them of a kind to identify the bacteria of human pyæmia with certainty. The latest author—Litten†—examined thirty-five instances of—as he calls them—septic diseases. His description proves them to have been what would commonly be called pyæmia. In all these instances bacterial emboli were invariably found in the centre of the metastatic deposits in the different organs. Their anatomical relationship clearly pointed them out as the starting-points of the secondary suppurations. Especially in the interior of the eye when involved in metastatic inflammation could the importance of the micro-organisms be clearly established. The bacteria were also found related to the minute hemorrhages so frequently observed in pyæmia. Generally an embolic plug of bacteria was found in the vessels from which the blood exuded—but not always. Litten speaks of micrococci-colonies almost wholly, but in some instances encountered also rod-shaped bacteria.—All observers admit that the place where bacteria—usually micrococci—can be most easily demonstrated is in the inflamed cardiac valves, since endocarditis is such a common lesion found in pyæmia.

*Orth, Martini, Heiberg, Litten and many others.

†Ueber septische Erkrankungen. Zeitschrift f. klin. Medizin, Vol. II, pp. 378 and 558.

Numerous have been the attempts to provoke pyæmia
experimentally in animals. But the older observations
can be passed over in silence. They have widened our
views of infectious diseases and have proven an incen-
tive to further work, but they were not accurate enough
to satisfy our present requirements. Many experiments
have been made by different parties ·in the hope of
obtaining pyæmia by the injection of putrid substances.
Since these substances contain many varieties of bacteria, variable and inconstant results were obtained.
Amongst other infectious diseases, true pyæmia did
sometimes appear in consequence of such injections,
but it was not even attempted to identify the corresponding parasites or to learn whether they were
specific in that disease. Again, in other instances
observers attempted to grow the bacteria taken from
pyæmic patients, outside of the body. But they
invariably chose as cultivating fluids Pasteur's or
Cohn's mineral solutions, in which pathogenic parasites cannot thrive at all. Hence the crop of bacteria
which they did get was really the progeny of germs,
unintentionally introduced. In spite of all precautions
to prevent the accidental access of foreign germs to
their flasks, these observers raised bacteria from
pyæmic pus, with no assurance that this pus—exposed
to the air—did not contain a variety of micro-organisms. When the blood was used for the inoculation
of the cultivating solution—as in the experiments of
Wolff*— negative results followed invariably, because
the mineral solution could not nourish the pathogenic
bacteria. Hence very little light was thrown upon the
etiology of pyæmia by such uncertain and conflicting
results.

The first definite statements as regards a well char-

*Virchow's Archiv, Vol. 81, p. 193.

acterized form of pyæmia in animals are those by
Koch.* He obtained in rabbits a disease characterized
by inflammation — and subsequently suppuration — at
the inoculated spot, with metastatic deposits in internal
organs, swelling of the spleen, and peritonitis. This
disease could be transmitted from one animal to
another by injection of the blood of the first victim.
Its original production was a matter of accident. In
a series of injections of putrid substances he got this
form of disease in one instance and could thence
transmit it to other animals. Its cause was found to
be the growth of a micrococcus in colonies in the
blood-vessels of the affected parts. The parasites
were quite small, about 0.25 micromillimeters in
diameter, and had a tendency to form thrombi in the
vessels. They spin around the blood corpuscles in a
characteristic manner and render them adhesive. Thus
the corpuscles adhere to each other and form thrombi,
from which fragments may be torn off by the blood-
current and carried along until they are caught in
some vessel too small to permit their passage. In
these embolic masses the micrococci continue to grow.
Since the micrococci are so readily arrested in the
vessels on account of their influence upon the adhe-
siveness of the corpuscles, they cannot exist in large
numbers in the circulating blood in spite of their
active growth. They were found, however, in the
fibrinous deposits on the surface of the abdominal
organs. No attempt was made to cultivate them
artificially. But their invariable presence in the disease, and their behavior in the causation of thrombosis
and embolism are sufficient proof that they produce
the disease. These results have since been fully confirmed by Semmer.†

---

*Traumatic Infective Diseases, p. 47.
†Centralblatt f. d. med. Wiss., 1881, No. 41.

It cannot be stated with certainty, whether there are different forms of pyæmia or not, due to different parasites. As has been mentioned before, Pasteur recognizes as the cause of pyæmia a short sausage-shaped "vibrio," exceedingly flexible and movable in its earlier stage, but later on motionless. He compares it to bacterium termo, like which it is constricted in its centre. It is evidently different from the micrococcus of Koch. Its injection under the skin produces abscesses. When these are numerous or large, it is apt to be carried along by the blood-current and deposited in internal organs, where it provokes secondary suppuration. The same result follows its direct introduction into the blood-vessels. But Pasteur lacks in precision both in the description of the micro-organism and—more so—of the morbid lesions. His paper* is really a mere sketch, which could hardly be accepted as conclusive, if published by any one not so favorably known in this department as Pasteur. It might seem from his researches, as if pyæmia could be produced by the entrance into the circulation of any parasite capable of causing suppuration. But in proof of the specific nature of the pyæmic virus, it must be remembered that the micrococcus found by Pasteur in furuncles proved harmless on injection into the blood-vessels. Yet in the same animals it caused suppuration when put under the skin. Acute abscesses also do not cause pyæmia when unopened, though Ogston found the corresponding micrococci in the blood. They were eliminated by the kidneys and could be seen in the urine without disease of the kidney. All experimental and clinical observations force upon us the view that pyæmia is produced by the presence of a specific micro-organism in the

---

*Moniteur Scientifique, 1878, p. 611.

blood-vessels, gaining entrance into the system through some wound.

DECOMPOSITION OF PUS.

We have shown above, that in wounds from which germs have been excluded the healing processes occur undisturbed. The entrance, however, of micro-organisms into the wound starts an irritation of its walls. Possibly there may be some forms of bacteria which do not irritate much if at all, for micrococci have been found, especially by Cheyne, in some aseptic wounds. If the only parasites present are the micrococci which produce suppuration, the struggle between them and the living animal cells ends in the victory of the latter. If the pus can only escape, the wound heals invariably, although slower than it would without such infection. But in wounds exposed to the air, or touched with impure instruments, other bacteria soon develop. According to the testimony of many observers such wounds may contain as great a variety of micro-organisms, as are found in any rotten fluid. The decomposition of the pus is the inevitable consequence of their presence. The energy of these putrefactive changes depends of course upon the relative number of bacteria present. This varies considerably. Whenever the pus or secretion of the open wound can drain off freely the bacteria are scant in number, while stagnating fluids teem with micro-organisms. Of course the mode of dressing is not without influence upon the growth of the bacteria. We do not know whether the putrefactive-bacteria exert a direct influence upon the exposed tissues. Even if that be not the case, the products of decomposition—which they engender—irritate the wound in an unmistakable manner. This reveals itself in redness and sensitiveness of the edges of the wound and in retardation of the healing process. The significance of the occurrence of putrefaction-bacteria in wounds can be best appreciated on comparing the healing of two abscesses, one opened in an aseptic manner, the other operated upon without such precautions. In both cases the micrococci of suppuration are present, but *these* parasites are always overpowered by the living tissues, if the pus can escape. Hence in the aseptic abscess the suppuration diminishes at once. as soon as it is opened. Indeed if it be opened at an advanced period, when the abscess is well circumscribed, and there remains no coccus-infiltration in the surrounding tissues, there occurs very little oozing of pus after the original contents have been evacuated. Without further pain the cavity is closed, in a time proportionate to its size. If no antiseptic precautions have been *intentionally* observed in the opening of the abscess, the course of it is always less favorable, though the exact history varies with the extent of the infection. In proportion to the number of putrefaction-bacteria and the decomposition to which they give rise, is the healing retarded. The suppuration is more profuse, and there is more tenderness of the wound, than in the aseptic case. and the duration of the regenerative process is always prolonged.

Moreover the presence of the putrefaction-bacteria is one of the factors in the causation of

TRAUMATIC FEVER.

The fever following wounds is no doubt engendered by different influences in different cases. A febrile disturbance may result from wounds kept perfectly aseptic by reason of a protective dressing, or on account of their subcutaneous position, as in simple

fractures. But this fever is very slight and can be
recognized only by means of the thermometer, and not
by any sensations of the patient. The cause of this
aseptic fever—as it has been termed by Volkmann and
Genzmer—is probably the re-absorption of products,
especially ferments, liberated through the mechanical
destruction of tissues. Experiments by Koehler, Edel-
burg and others have also shown, that the fibrin-fer-
ment set free during the coagulation of blood, can act
as a fever-producing agent. The fever from aseptic
wounds is never of long duration.

The prolonged fever following all extensive wounds
which do not pursue an aseptic course, is of a different significance. We do not know how far the micrococcus producing suppuration is reponsible for it. It
is true that when this parasite first invades the tissues
in the formation of an abscess, it causes a fever proportionate to the extent of the invasion. But this
fever ceases very quickly when pus can find free exit.

A more potent cause accounting for traumatic fever,
is the absorption of the products of decomposition
from the surface of the wound. It is indeed a common observation that the constitutional symptoms are
more marked, the more offensive the wound, and the
more imperfect the drainage of its secretion. Unlike
aseptic fever, the fever due to an impure wound *is*
accompanied by other disturbances, such as restless-
ness, want of appetite, and depression of spirits. It
is not claimed that these symptoms are due to the
entrance of bacteria into the blood. They can be produced in animals by the injection of the products of
putrefaction without the presence of micro-organisms.
Since the earlier experiments of Gaspard at the beginning of this century, numerous observers have studied
the effects of putrid material upon the body. But in

none of the earlier researches was there any distinction made between the *poisoning* with decomposed substances, and the *infection* due to the various forms of bacteria present in the putrid solution. Panum was the first to point out the difference in the nature of these two processes in 1855.*

PUTRID OR SEPTIC POISONING

can be produced with the products of decomposition of nitrogenous organic substances without the presence of living micro-organisms. In the experiments of Panum, in which macerations of rotten tissues were used, the solution was filtered by means of a suction pump through two layers of the finest Swedish filter paper, after which procedure the microscope could detect no bacteria in the filtrate. Culture experiments had not been used, hence doubts might be permitted whether a few isolated bacteria might not have passed through the filter. But in other experiments the absence of bacteria was fully guaranteed by eleven hours' continuous boiling of the infusion. By the boiling the strength of the poisonous fluid was reduced to about one-fifth of its original virulence, but this loss was probably caused by the adhesion of the poison itself to some flakes of albumen, which were coagulated by the heating. For the precipitated albumen proved intensely virulent on inoculation. The best criterion as to whether the symptoms resulting from the injection of the solution were those of poisoning or those of infection was the length of time elapsing until any consequences appeared. A chemical poison disturbs the functions of the tissues, as soon as it comes in contact with them, while a

* His researches were published originally in the Danish, and republished in 1874 in Virchow's Archiv., Vol. 60, p. 328.

struggle between the tissues and invading parasites becomes apparent only after the latter have multiplied to a sufficient extent. In the experiments of Panum there was no period of incubation. When enough of the putrid poison was introduced into the veins, death —preceded by convulsions and suffocation—was almost instantaneous, while the smallest quantity of the material capable of disturbing the animal system visibly, showed its effects within two hours, which period is far too short for any extensive multiplication of living beings. A medium dose produced the most characteristic symptoms of putrid poisoning, for while it did not kill too quickly to permit fair observation, the effects were of course more marked than from minimum doses, which did not preclude recovery. In these instances (in dogs) there occurred, within half an hour to two hours, an intense intestinal irritation, showing itself in severe vomiting and purging. This was accompanied by prostration and collapse. Characteristic, also, was the peculiar condition of the skin, which seemed too large for the animal, and could be gathered into folds, which remained for quite a time. When the animals recovered, these symptoms subsided slowly within twenty-four hours and were followed by very slow convalescence. In the fatal cases death came on in from four to twenty-four hours. The autopsy showed congestion of, and extravasation into, the lining membrane of the intestines, ecchymoses under the serous surfaces, and the blood in a black and fluid condition. The cadavers began to putrefy in a remarkably short time. The fatal dose of this poison was very small. Twenty-four centimeters of the putrid maceration necessary to kill a dog contained but seven centigrams solid residue, of which but an unknown portion could have been the poisonous substance.

These researches of Panum explain many of the symptoms observed in patients suffering from foul wounds. But they do not account for the most characteristic phenomenon—the fever. Panum did not find a rise of temperature the constant effect of his injections. But fever had been obtained in most of the experiments of the older French and German observers (Gaspard, Sedillot, and others; later on Billroth and Weber) in which various putrid fluids were introduced into the system. Though no attempt was made to exclude living germs in the former observations, the occurrence of fever within a *few hours* after the injection can only be attributed to the action of chemical poisons. The symptoms of putrid poisoning are by no means identical in the descriptions of different authors. The explanation of these discrepancies, however, is quite simple. The rotten material was not the same in all cases, and it was employed in widely different stages of putrefaction. The putrid poison is not a single chemical substance, it is a mixture of a number of unknown products. Thus Panum found, that on evaporating an alcoholic extract of his dried maceration-fluid, he could take up in water from this residue a substance, which produced a quiet sleep in a dog without further sickness.

Bergmann and Schmiedeberg* obtained from putrid yeast a crystalline base which they termed *Sepsin*. One centigram of this substance produced in dogs an immediate fever with the intestinal symptoms characteristic of putrid poisoning. But sepsin cannot be found in all putrid matter. Under Bergmann's guidance a number of his pupils† studied the various

---

*Centralblatt, 1868.

†Quoted by Hiller: Die Lehre von der Faeulniss, 1879. pp. 106 et seq.

conditions, under which poisons are produced by putrefaction, and the manifold symptoms they engender, but without determining the chemical nature of these complex substances.

A singular observation, made by all the experimenters, is the rapid decomposition of the cadavers of animals dead from putrid poisoning. This is likewise true of human corpses dead from blood poisoning. This fact has been quoted as an argument against the germ-theory and upon it have been based vague speculations to prove, that the presence of bacteria is merely a consequence of septic diseases. But it is the more conservative plan to admit that we cannot account for it satisfactorily as yet.

If the above-mentioned symptoms be really the effect of a chemical poison, which—unlike living parasites—cannot reproduce itself, it is to be inferred, that the blood of animals, suffering from putrid poisoning, is unable to transmit the disease to other animals, when injected in limited quantity. This was found to be true in the experiments of Gutman and Semmer.* A contrary observation, however, had previously been reported in a short communication by Hiller.† This author, believing the septic poison to be of the nature of a chemical ferment, attempted to extract it from dried rotten blood by means of glycerine, the solvent power of which for ferments is well known. The glycerine-extract produced in rabbits the symptoms of septic poisoning, viz: fever beginning with chills, diarrhœa, prostration, and emaciation leading to collapse and finally death. But the same train of symptoms could be reproduced by inoculating a second animal with the glycerine-extract of the *fresh* blood of

*Virchow's, Vol. 83, p. 99.
†Centralblatt f. Chirurgie, 1876, Nos. 14 and 15.

9

the first victim. Like other observers, to be referred
to later on, he found that the virulence of the blood
apparently increased in the animals successively injected, so that in the case of the tenth animal, or as it
might be called the tenth generation, $\frac{1}{100}$ of a drop of
the glycerine-extract proved fatal. But I am in doubt
whether these observations can really range as septic
poisoning. The claim, that an extraneous chemical
ferment can reproduce itself in the animal system, is
so opposed to our general knowledge, that it requires
a better substantiation in order to be accepted.
Though Hiller claims, that the microscope could
detect no bacteria in the glycerine extracts, I am not
satisfied that they were not there. For Koch has
since shown that it may be almost impossible to find
certain bacteria in the blood, except by the use of
staining methods. How much more difficult is hence
the detection of bacteria in a fluid possessing as high
an index of refraction as glycerine. Moreover Hiller
observed a period of incubation of several days at
first, though in the later generations this was reduced
to some hours. I would hence be more inclined to
consider the disease observed by Hiller to be a form
of real

SEPTICÆMIA.

It is scarcely possible to give at present an absolute definition of this disease. When it occurs as the
consequence of a foul wound, it appears simply as a
traumatic fever indefinitely prolonged, so that the
exact moment of its onset can not be stated. After
really aseptic wounds, on the other hand, it does not
occur. In other instances, in which the poison enters
the system through some slight wound, which had not
caused any traumatic fever, or in which the mode of

entrance of the virus cannot be traced, the disease begins with distinct chills. But then these latter cases amount always to a mixture of septicæmia with pyæmia, the so-called septico-pyæmia. In fact a pure uncomplicated septicæmia seems to be very rare in human pathology. Its symptoms are described as a more or less continuous fever with depression and prostration and often intestinal irritation. It cannot be said to be always fatal in man, though mostly so. The autopsy in the pure cases reveals nothing but swelling of the spleen. But in the majority of instances pyæmic changes, *i. e.* metastatic suppurations, are likewise found, showing that during life the distinction between the two diseases is scarcely possible in man. Yet there occur rare cases of blood-poisoning, which cannot be considered as *putrid poisoning*, because there is no wound with sufficient decomposition of the discharge to furnish the septic poison, while true pyæmia is excluded by the absence of metastatic deposits. These we cannot but consider as typical instances of septicæmia, however rare they may be. But I have not been able to find a single record of such a case in which either the presence or absence of bacteria was determined. The examination of the living blood would be insufficient, for during life pyæmia cannot be excluded with certainty. Moreover you will learn presently that in the experimental septicæmia of animals bacteria cannot always be found in the living circulating blood.

Many endeavors have been made to communicate human septicæmia to animals, but here as in pyæmia none of the results are really conclusive. Even if some of the observers did get septicæmia in their animals, they did not characterize it sufficiently in their description. Their only object was to see, whether the animals would get sick at all. But with material taken from other sources, *i. e.*, such as is furnished by rotten refuse of different kinds, several different diseases may be produced in animals, which all merit the name septicæmia. For by analogy with the corresponding disease of man, we can apply that term, whenever we meet with an infective fever continuing until death without other prominent symptoms, and characterized by the absence of all lesions, except swelling of the spleen. Moreover in the light of modern developments, we should restrict the term to those conditions in which bacteria are actually found in the blood. According to this definition we can recognize at least four different forms of septicæmia in animals due to different parasites of which I shall give the following synopsis:

I. Septicæmia due to very delicate bacilli, produced originally in the mouse by Koch.* These bacilli are about 0.8 to 1 micromillimeter in length, and about one-tenth as thick. They are so delicate, that they can be scarcely seen without staining. While growing they form dense masses, but never chains. Koch has seen spores in them occasionally. They have been cultivated later on by Koch and Loeffler† on the surface of a mixture of gelatine, peptone and meat-extract. The colonies, which they form on this substratum are characterized by a delicate arborescent shape. In the body of the infected animal they are found only within the blood-vessels. They often penetrate into the white corpuscles and multiply until the whole corpuscle forms but a cluster of bacilli. The inoculation of mice with these bacilli proves invariably fatal in from 40 to 70 hours—with a period of

*Traumatic Infective Diseases, p. 33.
†Mittheilungen aus dem Gesundheitsamte, p. 169.

incubation of about 24 hours. The disease can be transmitted to pigeons and sparrows, but not to field-mice. In the dog, cat, rabbit and white rat these bacteria provoke only a local inflammation resembling erysipelas.

II. Septicæmia due to oval micrococci, the greater diameter of which is about one micromillimeter. Koch* studied this form of disease first in rabbits, which are killed by these parasites in from 20 to 40 hours. No lesions were found after death but small scattered echymoses in different parts, and swelling of the spleen. Many small veins are choked with the micrococci and when they burst, allow the bacteria to extend into the tissues. This septicæmia could also be transmitted to mice.

III. Septicæmia produced by Koch and Gaffky† in rabbits and mice by means of a parasite too short to be called a bacillus, and too elongated to be termed coccus. These bacteria, about 1.4 by 0.7 micromillimeters in size, show an unstained central portion, when colored with aniline dyes, which gives them almost the appearance of a diplococcus although they have no central constriction. They show no active motion. They were cultivated in beef-broth or on the surface of a gelatine mixture containing meat infusion and peptone. On this substratum the colonies assume the form of characteristic globules. Rabbits are killed by them in 16 to 20 hours without other lesions than enlargement of the spleen and of the lymphatic glands. They neither plug the vessels, nor do they leave them and enter the tissues. The disease could be produced besides in bats and birds, while it was impossible to inoculate successfully guinea-pigs, white rats, cats and dogs.

*Loc. cit., p. 53.
†Mittheilungen, p. 93.

IV. A form of septicæmia obtained by Pasteur*
by inoculating rabbits with the saliva from a child
with hydrophobia. He called it at first a specific
" new disease," not being able to recognize it as
hydrophobia. But since it can be produced by the
saliva of many normal persons and possesses no other
characteristics it may just as well be termed septicæmia. The parasites appear in the form of a figure 8
about 0.5 micromillimeters in length, and are surrounded by a delicate halo. When cultivated in veal
broth they are slightly larger at first than in the
blood, and form chains, but resolve themselves after a
few days—to use the words of Pasteur—into small
round granulations. Gaffky supposes that this "new
disease" of Pasteur is identical with his septicæmia,
but on comparing the descriptions I find striking differences. Instead of Gaffky and Koch's negative
lesions, Pasteur found hemorrhages in the lungs, congestion and echymosis of the trachea, and local swelling and inflammation at the inoculated spot, besides
swelling of numerous lymph glands. The disease
killed rabbits in from eighteen to forty-eight hours.
It could not be transferred to pigeons (unlike Gaffky's septicæmia) or guinea-pigs. Probably the same
form of septicæmia has been studied by Sternberg†
of this country. He produced it likewise in rabbits
by the injection of human saliva, but found only the
saliva of some individuals—not of all—active. The
symptoms and lesions observed were identical with
those described by Pasteur. The description of the
micrococcus is more accurate, since Sternberg used
staining methods. It agrees on the whole also with
Pasteur's observation. The photographs published by

---

*Comptes Rendus, Vol. 92, p. 15.
†National Board of Health. Bulletin Apr. 30, 1881, No. 44.

Sternberg, although not very sharp, are different from those of Koch and Gaffky's septicæmia (form III.) The parasite could be cultivated in rabbits' bouillon or dogs' serum. It is not likely, that this completes the list of septi-cæmic diseases occurring 'in different animals. As long as we employ the term septicæmia with this provisional loose significance, we might include under this head all febrile affections not characterized by any localized symptoms or lesions and due to the pres-ence of some form of bacteria in the blood. Hence logically the term might even be applied to anthrax.

In the earlier researches on septicæmia it was sup-posed that the parasites causing the disease were identical with the bacteria of putrefaction. This view can no longer be sustained. The blood of the animal just dead of septicæmia teems with the characteristic micro-organisms, but gives no evidence of putrid decomposition. On the contrary it loses its virulence, when allowed to rot in the ordinary manner. While the fresh blood of the septicæmic animal can repro-duce the disease in almost incredible dilution, the occurrence of putrefaction soon deprives it of its spe-cific pathogenic property, and reduces its poisonous quality to that of ordinary rotten blood. Evidently the specific septicæmic bacteria are overpowered and crowded out of existence by the invasion of the same soil by the less dangerous organism of putrefaction. Sternberg found also, that virulent saliva could no longer produce septicæmia after it had undergone putrefaction. The non-identity of the septicæmic bac-teria and the common putrefactive forms is further shown by the inconstant results on inoculating animals with decomposing animal refuse. If the quantity injected be not large enough to kill speedily by septic poisoning, true septicæmia occurs only in a certain variable proportion of the experiments. The disease resulting may be either one of the above forms. But, when once produced, the disease can be transmitted indefinitely and with absolute certainty to further animals of the same or any other susceptible species. In those instances, in which the parasites were cultivated outside of the animal body, they retained all morphological and functional characteristics indefinitely and never changed into other forms, and never produced putrefaction of the soil in which they grew. All these facts harmonize only with the view that each form of septicæmia is produced by a separate and distinct parasite, not identical with putrefaction-bacteria, though found occasionally and accidentally in the same soil with the latter.

The blood of septicæmic animals possesses an astonishing degree of virulence. The infectious power of the blood is much greater than that of the original putrid material which served as the source of the virus. Coze and Feltz were the first to point out that the infectiousness of the virus seems to increase on being transmitted through a series of animals. This *progressive virulence* of the septicæmic "poison"—if we can use that term—attracted general attention, however, only after the striking experiments of Davaine reported to the French Academy of Medicine in the years 1872 and 1873. Davaine produced septicæmia by the inoculation of blood in a certain stage of decomposition. Like Koch later on he does not seem to have succeeded in every instance. But when once produced the disease could be transmitted indefinitely. It cannot be decided now, which of the above described forms of septicæmia, if any, Davaine observed. For very little reference was made by Davaine, or those

who confirmed his experiments, to the existence of
bacteria in the blood. It was simply stated that they
were there, but not which variety or in what number.

It must be remembered that staining methods were
not known at that time and that the delicate septicæmic
bacteria can be overlooked in the blood without them.
At any rate it was a disease fatal to rabbits in sixteen
to sixty hours without producing any lesions but
swelling of the spleen; and it could be transmitted to
guinea-pigs, mice and rats, but not to fowls and
pigeons.

On transmitting the disease from animal to animal
through twenty-five successive generations, it was found
that the dilution of the blood used for inoculation
could be continuously diminished without danger of
failure, until at last the one-thousand-millionth part
of a drop sufficed to kill a rabbit. This progressive
virulence was apparently confirmed in the subsequent
experiments of various French observers (Vulpian,
Bouley and others), of Clementi and Thin and of
Dreyer. But Koch has since pointed out, that the
"progressive virulence" is an unnecessary and un-
founded assumption. In his earlier experiments and
in his later researches with Gaffky it was learned that
the greatest possible virulence of the blood was
obtained in the second, or at the latest, the third
animal *successively* inoculated, in other words as soon
as the blood represents a "pure culture" of the parasite. In the first, and sometimes the second generation
of victims other bacteria are yet associated with the
specific parasites, but these non-pathogenic forms
introduced from the original source of the virus do
not persist in the blood of more than the first two
successive animals. At any rate he could not successfully employ a smaller quantity of blood for hypo-

dermic injection, when taken from any of the later generations than when obtained from the second, or at the most, the third animal. As he points out Davaine really admits the same truth in his own account of his researches, stating "that the septicæmic virus acquires immediately its greatest virulence." The alleged law of the progressive virulence of the septic blood is therefore a misinterpretation of the facts. In the researches of the other authors mentioned, who claimed to corroborate Davaine's discovery, there is no statement, whether they really tested the utmost extent of the virulence in the earlier generations.

It has been doubted whether the extreme virulence of septic blood in almost infinitesimal quantities could really be attributed to the bacteria found in it. But this query answers itself, when a well-stained specimen of blood is examined. It is evident in such a specimen that the parasites are many times more numerous than the red corpuscles. Now since animal blood contains over five millions of red corpuscles per cubic millimeter, and since one drop amounts to some thirty cubic millimeters, there are parasites enough present to account for the virulence of Davaine's minimal quantities.

There are several facts, however, in connection with septicæmia, which are as yet wholly unexplained. One of these is the harmlessness of the blood taken from the septicæmic animal before death. This was especially emphasized by Clementi and Thin as well as Dreyer in their repetitions of Davaine's experiments. They could reproduce the disease only with the blood taken from the animal at the moment of death, or within some hours after life was extinct. Koch does not seem to have tested this point, taking the blood used for inoculation only from the animal just dead. But Gaffky states that in one instance the blood proved virulent, though removed from a septicæmic rabbit two hours before the animal expired. The harmlessness of the blood during life indicates, that the parasites have not yet entered the circulating fluid. But the full explanation of this fact will only be possible after further studies. For up to the present all researches have really had no other object than merely to demonstrate that the disease is really due to parasites. No attempt has yet been made to study the behavior of the bacteria in the body.

More puzzling even is the fact, that the virulence of septic blood is not always destroyed by boiling. This was discovered by the French observers but more fully emphasized by Clementi and Thin. Quite recently it has again been confirmed by Rosenberger* who added further details. He experimented with the septicæmia of rabbits due to the short oval bacteria of Gaffky (form III). The virulence of the blood of the dead animal was much reduced by boiling, but not destroyed. On injecting the boiled blood in large quantity the original disease was reproduced and the blood of the animal, thus infected, was found to be as virulent, as that of any other septicæmic animal and contained the original form of bacteria. Yet Rosenberger claims that the heating destroyed the bacteria. For the infection of a sterilized meat-broth with a drop of fresh septicæmic blood produced a vigorous crop of the characteristic bacteria, while from the heated blood none could be cultivated. A similar paradoxical result was obtained by the same author in another infectious disease, which we shall discuss later on, viz: malignant œdema. This disease, characterized

*Centralblatt No. 4, 1882.

by the presence of an unmistakable bacillus growing
in the tissues can be produced by inoculating animals
with the serous effusion of a former victim. Here also
the virulence of the morbid fluid was reduced, though
not destroyed by boiling. Here also the bacilli were
apparently killed by heat, for they could not be cultivated outside of the body after boiling the fluid, and
yet they were reproduced in their characteristic forms
in an animal on inoculation with the boiled fluid.
The author attempts to explain these unexpected
results by denying the specific nature of the parasites
and attributing the cause of the disease to chemical
poisons, considering the bacteria only as associated
with, and not as productive of the disease. But this
explanation is a forced one and inadequate besides.
It seems to me more logical to admit, that such puzzling observations can only be explained by further
researches and not by speculative reasoning for which
the basis is yet wanting.

LECTURE VI.

Surgical Infections (continued).—Erysipelas.—Progressive Gangrene.—
Progressive Phlegmons.—Malignant Œdema.—Symptomatic Charbon (Quarter Evil).—Immunity from Intravenous Injection.—Tuberculosis: The Disease is Infectious.—The Bacillus Tuberculosis.—
Inoculation with the Isolated Bacilli.—The Mode of Spreading of
the Disease.—Methods of Staining the Bacilli.—The Significance of
their Presence in the Sputum.

ERYSIPELAS.

In this disease it was found some ten years ago by
Lukomsky,* that micrococci occur in the affected portion
of the skin and subcutaneous tissue. In sections
cleared with acetic acid, they were seen to plug the
lymphatic vessels. They were also met with outside
of them and in the blood-vessels, but this observation,
not in harmony with the more recent researches, is to
be accounted for by the fact, that his cases were
mostly complicated with other diseases. Various other
observations have since been published by different
authors (Billroth and Ehrlich, Tillmanns, Nepveu,
Bellien), which have not, however, added materially to

*Virchow's Archiv, Bd. 60, p. 418.

our knowledge, because they were not sufficiently systematic. But precise statements have appeared by Koch* and by Fehleisen.† Both have examined the skin of the cadaver as well as small pieces of skin snipped from the living patient. In all these instances‡ micrococci 0.3 to 0.4 micromillimeters in diameter were found, forming slightly curved chains. In stained sections it could be seen, that in a narrow zone just outside of the border of the erysipelatous redness, they grew in the lymphatic vessels and to a less extent in the interstices of the tissue. The infiltration extended in depth down to the subcutaneous tissue. This infiltration is evidently the forerunner of the erysipelatous process and precedes the inflammatory change by some hours. At the very edge of the disease, where the inflammatory changes are most active, the cocci are met with in still greater numbers. Here they exist all throughout the tissues and are found, also, in the interior of the round cells. But, as the centre from which the disease originated, is approached the parasites disappear completely. There is only one way of interpreting these observations. The parasites vegetate in the interior of the lymph vessels and lymph spaces and produce thereby an inflammatory reaction of the tissues which destroys them in turn. Some former observers, for instance Nepveu, have also found micrococci in the blood of erysipelas, but this was not corroborated by Fehleisen, when the blood was taken from the healthy parts.

Numerous attempts have been made to inoculate animals with erysipelas. Lukomsky,§ Orth‖ and Till-

*Mittheilungen, etc., p. 38.
†Deutche Zeitschrift f. Chirurgie. Bd. 16, p. 391.
‡Altogether five cadavers and bits of skin from sixteen living patients.
§Loco cito.
‖Archiv f. experimentelle Pathologie, Bd. I., S. 87.

manns* succeeded in only very few instances in producing erysipelas in rabbits with the contents of erysipelatous blisters in man. In most instances their
results were negative. The explanation of this uncertain effect is the absence or relative scarcity of the
parasites in the serum of the blisters. Their real
site is only in the lymphatic spaces. In other cases
again the faulty method was employed of trying to
grow the pathogenic bacteria in Pasteur's fluid which
cannot nourish them.

But all former uncertainty in transferring erysipelas
from man to animals loses its significance in view of
Fehleisen's† invariable success in reproducing the
disease by inoculation with the cultivated micrococci.
Excised bits of skin, removed of course with all precautions to avoid extraneous infection, were put into a
gelatinous solution of meat-extract and peptone and
kept at the proper temperature. There spread from
the implanted tissue a whitish growth, at first in the
form of scattered dots, coalescing afterwards to form
a delicate scum. This pure cultivation of the erysip-
elas-micrococci could be maintained—perhaps indefinitely—by transfer to a fresh soil. The parasites grew
as well on the surface of solidified blood serum, but
also even on potatoes. The inoculation of nine rabbits
reproduced the disease in eight instances, the ninth
animal possessing apparently an immunity. In thirty-
six to forty-eight hours fever began and a typical
erysipelas spread from the inoculated ear through a
variable part of the cutaneous surface. All the animals
recovered in from six to ten days. In one of the
rabbits the affected ear was amputated beyond the
border of the inflammation and the spread of the

---

*Archiv f. Klinische Chirurgie, Bd. 23, S. 437.
†Die Ætiologie des Erysipels, 1883.

disease checked thereby. Fehleisen has likewise successfully inoculated seven human individuals with erysipelas. His justification of this dangerous experiment was the old observation made by various surgeons, that sometimes tumors, which cannot be removed by the knife, disappear after an attack of erysipelas over that region. He seems to have accomplished that object in only one case definitely, viz.: a relapsing carcinoma of the breast. But while his other patients were not particularly benefited, none suffered any permanent harm. The micrococci which he employed for inoculation had been grown on solid soil for from four to seventeen generations. Some fifteen to sixty hours after the vaccination there occurred a chill, followed by fever, and coincident with it the typical erysipelas appeared, running thereupon its usual course. A second inoculation repeated inside of three months had no effect, while in one instance a spontaneous erysipelas which occurred a few months previously also frustrated the artificial infection. Fehleisen concludes, therefore, that an attack of erysipelas confers an immunity upon its victim which lasts some three months. Common observation indeed teaches that the immunity is not of long duration.

A disease closely resembling erysipelas in man can be produced in the rabbit also by means of another parasite. The minute bacilli which cause septicæmia (form I, p. 132) in mice, produce only a local reaction and not a constitutional disease in larger animals. In the cat, dog and rat the resulting inflammation is slight and of short duration. But in the rabbit these bacilli start a spreading inflammation of the skin attended with fever—only, however, if the inoculation is made in the ear or the cornea. In some few instances this leads to the death of the

animal. It is only in the severest attacks, that the
bacilli enter the blood; ordinarily they are confined to
the inflamed tissue. Loeffler,* who studied this form
of erysipelas, found it followed by a distinct immunity
against a second inoculation. Amongst thirty-three
rabbits he met with but two exceptions, and in these
cases an absolute immunity was granted by the second
attack. But this immunity does not follow the erysipelas, until after the lapse of some two or three weeks,
and during this time the inoculation may yet succeed
in a distant part, although ineffectual in the locality,
where it was first practised. In this curious instance
the "power of resistance" spreads gradually over the
cutaneous surface of the animal.

A third form of erysipelas has been observed,
though only in one instance, by Koch in his earlier
studies.† It was produced in the rabbit by a delicate
bacillus, larger, however, than the former one.

Of the other surgical infections occurring in man,
progressive phlegmons and hospital gangrene, the
bacterial origin has not yet been proven. But some
similar diseases have been studied experimentally in
animals by Koch. By inoculation with putrid blood he
obtained in some instances *a progressive destruction
of the tissues* in mice resembling hospital gangrene.‡
When once obtained it could be transferred from one
animal to another. Its cause was found to be the
vegetation of a micrococcus about half a micromillimeter in diameter, growing in chains. Its presence
proved destructive to the tissues even at some distance
beyond the vegetation, probably by the diffusion of
some poisonous product. Beyond the gangrenous

---

*Mittheilungen aus dem k. Gesundheitsamte, p. 169.
†Traumatic Infective Diseases, p. 56.
‡Traumatic Infective Diseases, p. 40.

10

portion the tissues were found in a violent state of inflammation.

In rabbits Koch* has studied a form of *spreading abscess* which seems quite common in these animals as I find a reference to it in the records of many other authors. The cheesy contents of these abscesses do not consist of pus, but of a finely granular material which does not take up aniline colors. A very small micrococcus measuring only 0.15 micromillimeters was found, however, in zoogloea masses on the walls of the abscesses and growing beyond into the tissues. This growth continues, until the death of the animal, which occurs within twelve to fifteen days. Koch considers the granular contents of the abscess to be the dead zoogloea masses. But since these contents are infectious to other animals he suspected the formation of spores, though he could not actually detect them. It must be remembered in this connection that spores have not yet been demonstrated in any other variety of micrococci.

In none of the instances of surgical infection thus described do we know how the contagion spreads. We can identify the parasites, we know that they will grow, if introduced into a wound and—what is the most valuable to us—we can exclude them by the strict antiseptic treatment of wounds. But we do not know yet, how they leave the body of one patient in order to reach another. As long as we cannot trace them thus in their migration, we cannot say with certainty, whether any one of these diseases is only infectious or also contagious in the ordinary sense of the word. For the clinical experience as regards the contagiousness of these affections is so ambiguous. that there exists as yet a diversity of opinion amongst

*Loco cito, p. 44.

surgeons. It is quite probable, that most, if not all, parasites causing the surgical infections, can vegetate outside of the body. The virus would therefore be both endogenous and ectogenous. At any rate the prevalence of these forms of bacteria and their frequent occurrence in putrid soils harboring a variety of forms, render this view plausible, though it has not yet been strictly proven, at least under the conditions actually occurring in nature.

Another disease, which might rank amongst the surgical infections, though perhaps not common in man, is

MALIGNANT ŒDEMA.

This disorder had previously been studied by Pasteur,* who called it septicæmia. But since the disease is characterized by a progressive œdema without the primary presence of the parasites in the blood, the name proposed by Koch,†—"Malignant Œdema,"— seems more appropriate. It is invariably fatal within twenty-four to forty-eight hours. From the point of inoculation there spreads pretty rapidly an effusion of reddish serum and at the autopsy the parasites are found abundantly in this fluid and in the tissues as far as the œdema goes. In larger animals very few, if any, occur in the blood, but in mice there are enough of them existing in the circulation, to render it impossible to distinguish this disease from anthrax. It has probably been mistaken for anthrax in many instances by former observers, which accounts for some inaccurate statements. The parasite is about the same length as the bacillus anthracis, but slightly thinner and possesses rounded ends. It is often, though not

---

*Bulletin of the Academy of Medicine, April 30th, 1878.
†Mittheilungen, etc.

always in a state of slight motion and, when it forms long filaments of coherent segments, the movements are serpentine.

Pasteur has cultivated this parasite in meat solution, but only in the absence of oxygen, for according to him it is anærobic and is killed by free oxygen, except when in the state of spores. Gaffky doubts this statement, as it can be found growing in the lungs of an infected mouse, where oxygen is not deficient. Still he could not cultivate it on the surface of gelatine, though he did grow it in the interior of boiled potatoes.

The spores of this bacillus are widely disseminated throughout nature. They are to be found in different waters, as well as in most of the surface soil, also occasionally in dust. These bacilli have also been found in the blood of strangulated animals on keeping the cadavers at a high temperature, evidently developed after death from pre-existing spores on some of the surfaces. We should hence expect this disease to be very common among susceptible animals, especially the rodents. But on the other hand, though the parasite exists almost everywhere, it cannot get a foothold in the system through a mere surface scratch. It is necessary to put it into the subcutaneous tissue in order to infect an animal, but with this precaution the success of the experiment is invariable. In the diseased tissues the signs of putrefaction are often present during life, viz.: a putrid odor and gas bubbles. But Gaffky has shown that this is a complication due to the presence of putrefaction-bacteria and that it may be avoided by inoculation with the isolated bacilli.

Two lamentable instances lately reported from the Berlin Medical Clinic by Brieger and Ehrlich[*] have

*Berliner Klinische Wochenschrift, No. 44, 1882.

taught us, that this parasite can also affect the human system. Two patients suffering from typhoid fever, and at the time in a state of collapse, received subcutaneous injections of tincture of musk. In both an œdema appeared at the spot of the injection on the thigh and spread up to the trunk, ending fatally without any augmentation of the existing fever. In the effused serosity the characteristic bacilli were found and identified by the successful inoculation of animals. The spores were probably contained in the tincture of musk, which through accident could. not be examined microscopically. But the same syringe and • bottle had been used on other patients without bad results. The authors suppose, therefore, that normally the human organism can withstand the attack of this parasite, but may lose its power of resistance when enfeebled by other causes.

It would be of importance to decide whether this disease—malignant œdema—is identical with an affection peculiar to cattle, viz.:

EMPHYSEMA INFECTIOSUM,

commonly known as the *Quarter Evil* or *Black Leg*, the *Rauschbrand* of the Germans, the *Charbon Symptomatique* of the French. As the latter name indicates, it has usually been mistaken for true charbon and indeed is even yet called anthrax fever. Its symptoms and the description of the parasites correspond with those of malignant œdema, but the identity can only be proven by actual experiment. It is essentially a progressive œdematous tumor with the presence of gas bubbles in the effusion and is almost always fatal. In the serosity a rod-shaped parasite has been found by Feser. But the closest study of .

it has been made by Arloing, Cornevin and Thomas
in numerous communications to the French Academy
of Sciences since 1880. Like the parasites of malignant œdema, the bacteria of this disease resemble the
bacillus anthracis, but have rounded ends and possess
an unmistakably active motion. Sometimes a clear
granule is seen at one end, perhaps a spore. These
rods are found in the interior of the emphysematous
tumor, in the lymphatic glands, and to a less extent in
the viscera. Very few are seen in the blood, but
some ovoid brilliant corpuscles, isolated, or joined in
twos or threes, were met with in the circulating fluid.
The significance of the latter was not determined.

For inoculating purposes Arloing, Cornevin and
Thomas used the fluid obtained by bruising the
emphysematous tissues. They do not seem to have
cultivated the parasites outside of the body. The disease could be transferred to cattle and sheep, guinea-
pigs and rabbits. In rats only local gangrene · was
caused without fatal issue. Dogs and fowls proved
insusceptible. Like in malignant œdema, it was necessary to put the parasites deep into the tissues; they
could not enter through surface wounds. Inoculation
with a minute quantity produced sometimes only
slight local symptoms without death. Of the most
interest are the studies of the French authors on
intravenous injection of the parasite. The fluid used
was deprived of all other grosser particles by filtration. The intravenous injection gave rise to a slight
temporary fever and sickness, but by itself never
proved fatal. But if an extravasion of blood is caused
during this time by some contusion, the bacilli
develop in the tissues and produce the usual localization, terminating fatally. If this accident does not
happen, the intravenous injection is not dangerous to

life, but confers absolute immunity upon the animals
against subsequent inoculation in the tissues. In
several series of public experiments Arloing, Cornevin
and Thomas have demonstrated that cattle and sheep
can thus be protected against the disease.

A more convenient method, however, for protective
inoculation was obtained by attenuating the virus and
then injecting it hypodermically. The fluid containing the parasites is dried at 32° C., and the residue
taken up by twice the amount of water. This mixture
is then kept at 100° C., during six hours. Another
portion similarly treated, but heated only up to 85°
C., is used for a second inoculation eight days later
to render the comparative immunity absolute. The
authors state, that the parasites contained spores before
they were heated, and indeed it seemed very unlikely,
that the developed bacilli could withstand this high
temperature. At any rate it is a fact of much interest, that the virulence of spores also may be modified
by such treatment. The virus thus mitigated may yet
prove dangerous, if used too freely, but a subcutaneous
injection of one centigram (of the dry material) for
sheep, and two or three times that amount for cattle,
just suffices for protection without risk from the
vaccination itself.

Another method of attenuating the virus has been
proposed by Nocard and Mollereau.* It consists in
the action of oxygenated water (peroxide of hydrogen). When mixed with oxygenated water the parasite is killed after the lapse of some hours, but prior
to its death passes through all stages of diminished
virulence. When enfeebled so far as not to cause the
death of an animal, it gives the latter a comparative
immunity, which can be rendered absolute by repeated

---

*Bulletin of the Academy of Medicine, Jan. 2nd, 1883.

inoculation with a stronger virus. The communication is so far principally of theoretical interest in showing the effect of oxygen in its active form upon micro-organisms. Practically this method has only been tested upon some guinea-pigs and one goat.

TUBERCULOSIS.

Seldom, if ever, has any medical discovery been received immediately with such intense interest as the modest announcement by Robert Koch* within the past year, that he had traced tuberculosis to the presence of a bacterial parasite. And yet the ground had been fully broken for this discovery, it was recognized by all competent pathologists, that this is an infectious disease and attempts had even been made by others to demonstrate the parasite presumably the cause of tuberculosis. But while these previous researches could not command universal respect on account of their want of precision, Koch's statements were . so positive and his high reputation gave them such a speedy circulation, as to provoke a remarkable enthusiasm, but, on the other hand also some bigoted opposition.

Since Villemin showed in 1865 that tuberculosis is inoculable in the lower animals by means of products of the disease, this statement has been completely confirmed by all other experimenters. In susceptible animals, like rabbits and guinea-pigs, the introduction of tubercular nodules, or of pus from tuberculous inflammation, into any part of the body invariably results in the eruption of tubercles at that spot and very often also in the production of a general tuberculosis of internal organs. In other animals . not so liable to take the disease spontaneously, as cat and

---

*Berliner Klinische Wochenschrift No. 15, Apr. 10, 1882.

dog, its experimental production is not so certain to succeed, unless large quantities of tubercular material are used and are implanted into the interior of the body. But it has been claimed that tuberculosis will also result in rabbits from inoculation with non-tubercular matter, or from the simple introduction of foreign bodies under the skin. If this were true it would denote that no "specific virus" is requisite in order to originate tuberculosis. Such an important claim should therefore receive due critical attention. As regards the fact itself there can be no doubt. Numerous observers have seen animals become tuberculous after placing setons, or bits of glass or wood under the skin. But rabbits and guinea-pigs contract this disease often, even without such apparent cause, especially in close confinement and when kept in laboratories in which experiments have been made upon tuberculosis. Thus Formad* who has lately referred to this point, found most of his animals tuberculous in a previous study upon diphtheria.† If this is hence such a common disease in his laboratory and stables, there is nothing surprising in the fact, that amongst the animals inoculated with material of non-tubercular origin many should also take the disease. But in localities, where tuberculosis does not prevail amongst the animals, the effects of inoculation are evident and not at all ambiguous. Under those circumstances while every rabbit, which is infected purposely gets tuberculous, the disease does not appear after simple wounds or the introduction of foreign bodies. The study of tubercular infection in a locality, thoroughly infected with the disease is as difficult and unsatisfactory, as would be a research on

---

*Philadelphia Med. Times, Nov. 18, 1882.
†National Board of Health Bulletin, Supplement No. 17, 1882.

the virus of small-pox during an epidemic of that affection. Every unprotected individual inoculated with variolous crust would be sure to take small-pox, but a great many, who received injection of some harmless material, might also be stricken with the disease, because the virus would be disseminated through the air, as well as by the lancet of the experimenter. Cohnheim and Fraenkel, who found every animal tuberculous in the laboratory of the Berlin pathological institute, no matter how slight had been the wound previously inflicted, got the disease only, when they purposely produced it by proper infection, on repeating these experiments in their separate private dwellings. Now it may seem strange to medical men that tuberculosis is so infectious and can be communicated so easily unintentionally through the air or the cage of the animal, for such is not the experience as far as man is concerned. But it is true, nevertheless, of rodents. All animals are not equally susceptible to tuberculosis or any other disease.

Even in infected localities the specific nature of the tubercular virus can be proven by inoculation in parts, where the disease does not localize itself spontaneously. The eye according to all observers is very rarely, if ever, the seat of tuberculosis in animals. But in the hands of numerous observers* the introduction of tubercular material into the anterior chamber of the eye never failed to produce tuberculosis of the iris. Other fluids or solid fragments, not of tuber-

---

*Cohnheim, Die Tuberculose vom Standpunkte der Infectionslehre, 1879.—P. Haensell, Archiv f. Ophthalm. Bd. XXV, H. 4, p. 1.—Deutschmann, ibidem, p. 280, and Bd. XXVI, H 2, p. 99.—A. Costa Pruneda, ibid., Bd. XXVI, H. 3, p. 174.—Salomonsen, Nordisk Medicinsk Archiv., 1879, No. 19.—Samuelsohn, Bericht d. Heidelberger Gesellschaft, in Centralblatt f. Augenheilkunde, Feb. 1880.—Baumgarten, Centralblatt f. d. med. Wiss., 1881, No. 15.—Schuchard, Virchow's Archiv, Vol. 88, p. 28.

cular origin, may destroy the eye by suppurative
inflammation, when put into the anterior chamber, but
they never start a tubercular process. In properly
executed experiments with tubercular material there
results a slight temporary—if any—inflammation. But
after the lapse of some twelve days the guinea-pig*
thus inoculated invariably shows an eruption of gray
nodules in the iris, which gradually coalesce and
destroy the eyeball. Gross appearances, as well as the
microscope, characterize this process as tuberculosis.
In most, though not all instances, general tuberculosis
of other organs follows in the course of some weeks.
Sometimes, however, the process remains localized. In
either case the nature of the disease is the same, but
in the latter instance the resistance of the animal to
the tubercular invasion is greater. No matter whether
the disease remains localized or becomes disseminated
throughout the system, the virus is the same, only
the reaction of the animal varies.

Indeed, all of the numerous recent researches, conducted with proper care, lead to the conclusion, that
the best criterion of the tubercular nature of any
morbid process is the inoculabilty of the products.
Whatever can reproduce tubercle on inoculation, contains the tubercular virus and is tubercle. The
structure of the morbid products is by means as
characteristic of the nature of the disease as their infectiousness, for notable differences occur in the amount
of reticulum of the tubercular nodule, in the presence or absence of giant-cells and even in the
general architecture of the disease-growth in different
animal species and even in the different organs of one
and the same animal. Thus the pearl-tumors of cattle
are so different in their structure from tubercles in

---

*15 to 20 days in the rabbit.

man and other animals, that the microscope alone could
not decide on their tubercular nature.   But inoculation-
experiments prove their identity.   It has furthermore
been shown in such experiments by Cohnheim and by
Schueller,* that we must range amongst the localized
tubercular processes not only the chronic inflammation of joints, as had previously been claimed, but
also the scrofulous lymph-glands and lupus.

The nature of the tubercular virus was first investigated by Klebs† and by his pupil Reinstadler.‡   The
assumption, that it was constituted by bacteria was
tested by culture-experiments in albumen, in which
the growth of granules and mobile short rods was
observed.   There can be no doubt now, since Koch's
latest researches, that *the* bacilli, really the cause of
tuberculosis, were not seen at all by these authors, for
they could not have grown under the circumstances.
Still it was claimed by Klebs, that he reproduced the
disease with the cultivated parasites.   No satisfactory
explanation can be given of such results, which are
undoubtedly erroneous, except that the material used
for inoculation still contained some of the true tubercle-bacilli, which the author overlooked in the absence
of staining methods, or that unintentional infection
occurred through insufficient disinfection of the instruments.   Schueller claims to have corroborated Klebs'
investigation, but to his own experiments the same
criticism applies, as well as to those of Toussaint,§
who seeks the cause of the disease in a micrococcus.
At any rate the methods employed by these authors

*Experimentelle und histolog. Untersuchungen ueber d. Entstehung
u. Ursachen d. skrophuloesen n. tuberculoesen Gelenkleiden, 1880.

†Communication to the Congress of German Naturalists at Munich,
1877.

‡Archiv f. experiment Pathologie Bd. 11, p. 103.

§Comptes Rendus, 1881.

seem altogether insufficient, when compared with the preciseness displayed and the spirit of severe criticism exercised by Koch in his celebrated publication.* More accurate, undoubtedly, was the observation of Baumgarten,† who saw in all tubercular nodules bacilli evidently identical with those Koch described at the same time. But this author did not go beyond their detection, he did not demonstrate their importance.

The bacilli, which Koch discovered can be recognized only with great difficulty without staining, on account of their delicacy and minuteness. Since they cannot be rendered visible at all by the ordinary methods of staining, we can readily understand why they had not been previously seen (except by Baumgarten, who treated the sections with caustic potash solution). The special method, which Koch used for their detection we shall describe later on in connection with the examination of the sputum. The bacilli thus stained appear as slender rods one quarter or half as long as a red blood-corpuscle, and extremely thin. They can be identified with greater certainty by means of their behavior to aniline colors, rather than by their shape and size alone. For with the exception of the bacilli of leprosy, from which they differ in shape, no other bacteria have as yet been found, which possess the same peculiarities with reference to staining. When examined fresh, these never show any active movements. These parasites are found most abundant at the border of any progressive tubercular infiltration, partly in the interior of cells, partly free between them, but they exist also throughout the entire tubercular growth, though to a less extent. Their number is in some proportion to the activity of

*Berliner Klin. Wochenschrift, No. 15, 1882.
†Centralblatt f. d. med. Wissenschaften, No. 15, 1882

the morbid process. When the latter is arrested, very few bacilli can be found. The imperfect staining of these few indicates, that they are dead. Wherever giant-cells occur, they contain some bacilli in their interior, though here also the parasites may disappear by disintegration. Not infrequently the bacilli appear granular and contain from two to four oval spores. The importance of these micro-organisms with reference to tuberculosis is evident, when we learn that Koch found them in every instance in the examination of eleven cases of human miliary tuberculosis, twelve of caseous bronchitis, one of tubercle of the brain, two of intestinal tuberculosis, three of scrofulous glands and four instances of fungous arthritis of man. They were never missed in ten cases of pearl-disease of cattle, some two dozen different animals dead of spontaneous tuberculosis and about 200 animals inoculated with the disease. Koch's researches have been made on such an extensive scale, that the confirmation by other authors,* of the invariable presence of these bacilli in the tubercular products can hardly add any more to their conclusiveness.

The *bacillus tubercnsis* has been cultivated by Koch on the surface of solidified blood-serum. The tubercular nodules from fresh internal organs of animals and of man were placed on this soil, whereupon the colonies of bacilli in their interior kept on growing and gradually extended in the form of white scales over the surface of the serum. The growth is very slow. so that it requires about ten days before it is at all apparent. The slow growth and the dryness of these scales distinguish such a pure culture from all other bacteria. Moreover the growth is *limited to a*

---

*Ehrlich, Sternberg, Balmer and Fraentzel, Gibbes, Williams, Lichtheim and others.

temperature of 30 to 41° C. In the course of several weeks the growth of a colony was completed, but the cultivation was continued by transferring a fragment of this first culture to a fresh soil. The parasite could thus be grown for months without any change in its properties.

The inoculation of animals with the isolated parasites did not fail to produce tuberculosis in a single instance out of some two hundred experiments. The effect was the same, no matter how long the bacilli had been cultivated outside of the animal body. In some instances this was continued for some 140 days. Injection of the isolated parasites into the anterior chamber of the eye, into the peritoneal cavity, into the blood-vessels or simply under the skin, rendered every animal tubercular, not only the susceptible rabbits and guinea-pigs, but also the more resistant rats, cats and dogs. In the less susceptible animals, however, it was requisite to put the parasites into some protected locality, like those mentioned. The mere inoculation of superficial wounds did not suffice, for on account of the slow growth of the tubercle-bacilli, they cannot gain a foothold through surface abrasions, but are eliminated. The infection with the isolated parasites leads to quicker and more extensive results, than when the crude tubercular material is employed, on account of the greater number of bacilli in the former case. In all of Koch's experiments the originally localized disease was followed by disseminated tuberculosis. There is always a tubercular infiltration and later on ulceration at the site of the infection, from which the disease then spreads to the rest of the system.

The manner, in which the disease spreads most commonly in man, is assumed by Koch to be the fol-

lowing: The sputum of most consumptives contains
the bacilli. However readily the developed bacilli
may succumb to the influence of time, desiccation or
damaging agents, the spores, which are often, though
not invariably, contained in the sputa, share the inde-
structibility of bacterial spores in general. The drying
of the expectorated matter and its subsequent conversion into dust by the foot, that treads on it, or any
other force, disseminates these spores throughout the
atmosphere. Whenever they settle on a suitable soil
the bacilli develop. We are evidently exposed to this
infectious dust in all localities where consumptives have
ever lived and expectorated, i. e., all over the civilized
world. It reaches the interior of the lungs and if it
can find the proper conditions for development, its
growth begins. That sputum does retain its infectiousness on drying, Koch proved by inoculating animals successfully with material dried since eight weeks.
The experiments of Tappeiner* on the other hand had
previously shown, that the inhalation of tubercular
matter, for instance, a spray of an emulsion of sputum,
does lead, invariably, to the infection of the animal,
even in the more resistant dogs. Finally the evidence
seems complete, when we remember that the disease is
always localized primarily at the point of infection
and that in the great majority of instances tuberculosis begins in the lungs. But Koch does not claim
that this is the only mode of the dissemination of the
disease. Ransome† has found micro-organisms in the
condensed breath of consumptives, which gave the
color-reaction of the bacillus tuberculosis. But the
number, thus exhaled, must be small compared with

---

* Communication to the German Congress of Naturalists at
Munich, 1877.

† British Medical Journal, Dec. 16, 1882.

the large amount of bacilli in the sputum. The disease besides can be communicated by the consumption of tubercular material, as has been proven in animals by quite a number of different observers. In such instances it begins in the intestines or mesenteric glands. It is not probable, that the virus can multiply outside of the animal body, on account of the high temperature it requires, the complicated nourishment it needs, and the slow growth even under the most favorable circumstances.

Koch's researches have as yet received no adequate confirmation. Korab* claims to have cultivated the bacilli and inoculated animals with them successfully, but does not state any details. His object was to prove the destructive properties of Helenin on the tubercle parasites. Sternberg† had but partial success in the repetition of Koch's works, but admits the incompleteness of his own researches. The mere presence of the parasite in tubercular products has been confirmed by all observers. On the other hand objections mostly of a speculative nature have been urged against Koch's work, none of them, however, founded on actual observation. The query, raised by some authors as to the bacterial nature of the bacilli, has no sense at all in view of their easy demonstration. Formad has recalled the old time-worn arguments of the occurrence of tuberculosis in animals without "specific" infection, but has ignored that others have trodden the same ground before him and have been completely refuted. At any rate no one has yet shown, that the disease can ever exist without the presence of the bacillus tuberculosis.‡

---

*Comptes Rendus, No. 10. Vol. 95, 1882.

†Medical News, Nov. 18, 1882.

‡While these lectures go to press an important confirmation of

11

Apart from the fundamental scientific importance of Koch's work, it has almost at once led to immediate practical results. Koch's own statement, that the bacilli are often present in the sputum of consumptives, has been confirmed by a host of other observers, so that the microscopic examination of the sputum possesses now a decided diagnostic value.* It is necessary hence to become acquainted with the mode of demonstrating the bacilli.

The tubercle bacilli do not take up the ordinary aniline colors readily. They require some "mordant" to fix the dye on them, but when once stained, they hold the color more tenaciously than other bacteria or animal cells. Koch's original staining method required the use of a solution of methyl blue (one part concentrated alcoholic solution in 200 parts of water) with the addition of $\frac{1}{10000}$ part of potassic hydrate or some other alkali. Specimens were kept in it for twenty-four hours, which time could be shortened by heating gently. By means of a concentrated filtered solution of Vesuvin in water, the blue color was then removed from all structural elements but the bacilli, which now appeared blue on a brown ground. This method seems tedious and not easy to employ. Ehrlich[†] has

---

Koch's work has just appeared by Watson Cheyne. In a preliminary report (Lancet, March 17th, 1883) to the "Association for the Advancement of Medicine by Research," he states, that he has tested the virulence of pure cultures of the alleged parasites of tuberculosis, received personally from Toussaint and from Koch. The former material, containing micrococci, was found absolutely inert, though Toussaint had rendered animals tubercular by inoculation with it. This result Cheyne refers to a gross self-deception due to insufficient disinfection of the syringe employed, as well as of the locality, in which the animals were kept. On proper attention to the hygiene of the animals and the disinfection by heat of all the utensils, Cheyne found that no animal ever

*Vide Gradle and Woltmann, Philadelphia Med. News, Feb. 17, 1883.
†Deutsche Med. Wochenschrift, No. 19, 1882.

since substituted aniline oil or "crude aniline" as a mordant for the alkali with the use of fuchsin as the first color. The specimen is then decolorized in nitric acid diluted with twice the amount of water, until all visible color has just left it, whereupon it is washed. Again the tubercle bacilli are the last elements to yield their tint, but their detection is facilitated by restaining the ground blue. They now appear as ruby red rods on a blue ground. In the case of sputum a minute particle is spread and dried in a thin film upon a cover glass and the film thereupon hardened by passing it through a flame. An instantaneous staining can now be accomplished by placing it in a watch glass filled with the solution and heating, until it simmers. The experience of different authors has shown this to be the quickest way to prepare the solution, viz: to dissolve aniline oil in water, to filter and to keep on hand, and to add to a watch-glassful of this fluid some eight drops of a saturated alcoholic solution of fuchsin. The specimen is then decolorized as above described. Gibbes* has suggested the addition of more alcohol to this fluid in order to keep it stable, but I have had the neatest result with a modification of Ehrlich's process which I have published with Mr. Woltmann in the "Medical News."† Two grams of fuchsin are dissolved in a

became tuberculous, except when purposely infected with Koch's bacilli, or material containing them. The animals, which had become infected with true tuberculosis in the hands of Toussaint, showed the usual abundance of Koch's bacilli, in the tubercular organs, but no micrococci. Twenty-five rabbits received foreign substances, under the skin, in the anterior chamber of the eye and in the peritoneal cavity, of which not one became tubercular, because they were kept in healthy stables. Koch's statements on the other hand Cheyne was able to confirm word by word as regards the appearance and color-reaction of the bacilli,

*Lancet, Aug. 5, 1882.
†Feb'y 17, 1883.

mixture of five grams aniline oil and twenty grams of alcohol, to which twenty grams of water are gradually added. This fluid, once filtered, can be kept as stock, but I have since found, that it will not remain clear for more than three or four weeks. For use it is simply diluted with twenty or thirty times as much water and the specimen kept in it at least two hours. A warmth of 40° to 60° C. favors the staining, but when the bacilli are few in number, they are apt to be overlooked unless a very deep color is imparted to them by an exposure up to twenty-four hours. Hereupon it is decolorized in dilute nitric acid, washed and the ground stained by dropping on a two per cent. solution of aniline blue and washing again after one minute's exposure. It can now be examined at once in water or mounted permanently in Canada balsam. The detection of isolated bacilli in such a specimen is quite difficult without an Abbe's condensor, but with its use they can scarcely be overlooked. Still I have assured myself, that an insufficient staining will allow the bacilli, if few in number, to escape detection and I consider it best, therefore, to deepen the color as much as possible in the examination of sputum for diagnostic purposes. It seems most plausible to me, that those observers (Guttmann, perhaps also Pfeiffer)

---

their distribution in the disease, their cultivation and virulence. He adds, furthermore, the different forms in which the disease appears clinically depend on the variable resistance of the individual to the parasitic invasion. Whenever the parasites can vegetate luxuriantly, the disease appears as catarrhal pneumonia rapidly destructive to the lung tissue, while the slower forms of fibrous pneumonia remain localized for a time on account of the production of a barrier of granulation tissue around the tubercular nodules, which hinders the further spreading of the bacilli from the affected spot. According to Cheyne the bacilli grow primarily in the interior of the alveolar epithelial cells, the proliferation of which forms the essential basis of the tubercular nodule. He could trace the giant cells to a coalescence of separate epithelial cells. Hence

who missed the bacilli relatively often in the sputum of consumptives, did not stain their specimens sufficiently. I say this with more confidence, since I have become acquainted with another method, which stains the bacilli so deeply, that it is impossible to overlook them.

The mordant, used in this case is carbolic acid, to a five per cent. aqueous solution of which is added about one fifth or eighth the quantity of a saturated alcoholic solution of fuchsin. The fluid precipitates some of the dye on standing, hence it is preferable to mix the two constituents at the time when required, no filtering being necessary. The dried sputum is allowed to float in this fluid, or a drop of it is simply placed on the film of the cover-glass. The staining does not require a full minute, if the specimen be heated. But the heat must not reach the boiling point and, when once stained, the specimen cannot be again exposed to heat without damage. The bacilli, thus treated, do not retain the color quite as tenaciously, as when stained with the aniline method, hence a little more caution is requisite, while decolorizing with nitric acid. But on the other hand the tint given to the bacilli is so intense, that there is no object to restain the ground with a contrasting color. Even without a condenser the bacilli, though

according to him the starting point of the disease in pulmonary phthisis is the alveolar surface, and the spreading of the process is partly due to the continued vegetation of the bacilli in extending from each center, partly to the infection of fresh alveoli, by mechanical transfer of the sputum.

Another publication lately issued is by Spina (Studien ueber Tuberculose, 1883). It claims to be a complete refutation of Koch's work. Spina finds the tubercle bacilli not characterized by any color-reaction, fails to detect them in the tubercles of interior organs and obtains no characteristic result from inoculation with the cultivated micro-organisms. But as Koch has justly said in a reply (Deutsche Med. Wochen-

there be but one in the field, attract the eye immediately. Since the application of this method does not consume more than three or five minutes, and the material requisite is so conveniently procured, I would recommend it most for the clinical examination of sputum. But it has this drawback. With the aniline method or Koch's original procedure the difference in the reaction of the tubercle-bacilli and other bacteria is absolute, while on staining by means of the carbolated solution the difference is only relative. While the tubercle-bacilli are the last elements to yield their color to the acid, still they too begin to fade, when some other kinds of bacteria have not yet had all their color abstracted by the acid. Hence there may be some stained bacteria left in the specimen. I found in most sputa a micrococcus in chains and a bacillus a trifle longer and much thicker than the real tubercle-bacilli. The latter, however, are stained much darker and can be recognized besides by their shape and size. While therefore this method enables us to decide instantly, whether the sought for bacilli are absent in a sputum, any doubt as to their identity in case of their presence may be removed by the use of the more characteristic aniline method. The bacilli, thus stained in the sputum, are of the appearance above described, the rods being often curved or two of them forming a figure V. Frequently they are granular on account of the spores they contain, which spores are distinctly stained. Sometimes irregular groups of spores are seen. The bacilli may be very

---

schrift, No. 10, 1863), Spina's experiments are but a caricature of his own. He shows a want of familiarity with staining and examining methods, his cultivating soil was not in a proper condition and the inoculation experiments were performed on *two* rabbits. What a contrast between such hasty work and Koch's researches extending over two years and involving over 200 different animals!

few in number, perhaps only one in several fields of
the microscope, or on the other hand a few dozen
may be found in every field with a power of 500 to
900 diameters. When numerous they form small
groups, otherwise they are scattered throughout the
field.

Koch's original statement, that the tubercle-bacilli
are often present in the sputum of consumptives ha
been fully confirmed by the published observations of
some fifteen to twenty different authors, while no
voice has as yet been heard to the contrary. These
same authors have all examined some few—or in other
cases, quite a number—of specimens of sputa from
other non-tuberculous diseases, without finding these
bacilli. This accumulated evidence, based on the negative results of at least 150 to 200 examinations of
non-tuberculous cases, proves absolutely, *that the presence of the characteristic tubercle-bacilli in the sputum
indicates pulmonary tuberculosis.* When they are
present, there can be no question as to the existence
of the disease. But are they invariably present? The
claims of different authors do not all agree on this
point. Guttmann* examined one hundred slides, in
one fourth of which only the parasites could be found.
He does not state how many different cases these
specimens represent. From his own description I
infer, that he did not stain for a sufficient length of
time and hence overlooked the imperfectly colored
bacteria in many instances.

Pfeiffer† examined daily the sputa of four patients
during twenty-five days. In the mildest case the
bacilli were found in all but seven slides, in the
severest instances they were missed only three times.

*Berliner Klin. Wochenschrift, No. 52, 1882.
†Berliner Klin. Wochenschrift, No. 3, 1883.

Altogether they were absent sixteen times out of one hundred examinations. Even in this case I suspect they were overlooked occasionally, since Pfeiffer used at first gentian-violet for staining, and only later the deeper color of fuchsin. On the other hand they were found *every time* by Ehrlich[*] in 26 phthisical patients, by Gibbes[†] in 19 instances, by Balmer and Fraentzel[‡] in 120 consumptives, by Ziehl[§] in 73 cases, by D'Espine[||] in 20 patients, by Heron[¶] in 62 cases, by West (a) in 50 instances, by Wipham (b) in 20 consumptives, by Dreschfeld(c) in 46 consumptives, and by myself (in conjunction with Mr. Woltmann) in some thirty to thirty-five consecutive tubercular patients. But it is not always evident in the publications quoted, whether they were encountered at every examination of one and the same patient. Balmer and Fraentzel insist on repeating the search for the bacilli at least on three different days, in case they are not seen the first time. Lichtheim (d) also claims to have detected them in every case, though not on every examination. He does not say how often. In our experience we have never examined any specimen of sputum in vain, if bacilli were found at any time in the expectoration of that patient, provided only the staining was sufficient. Still I have just searched three times for the bacilli without being certain of their presence, in the sputum of a patient

---

*Deutsche Med. Wochenschrift, No. 19, 1882.
†Lancet, Aug. 5th, 1882.
‡Berliner Klin. Wochenschrift, No. 45, 1882.
§Deutsche Med. Wochenshrift, No. 5, 1883.
||Quoted in Lancet, Jan. 13, 1883.
¶Lancet, Feb. 3rd, 1883.
(a) Lancet, Feb. 10th, 1883.
(b) Lancet, Feb. 10, 1883.
(c) British Med. Journal, Feb. 17th, 1883.
(d) Fortschritte der Medicin, No. 1, 1883.

dying of a rapid catarrhal pneumonia, though no
autopsy could be performed to confirm the diagnosis.
Dettweiler and Meissen* also saw two cases,—as they
say—of unmistakable phthisis, out of eighty-seven
patients in the sputum of which the bacilli were not
detected. Reviewing this evidence, therefore, we can
assert, that the bacilli can be found in the sputum of
the overwhelming majority of phthisical patients, certainly over ninety, if not ninety-five per cent., and that
in most cases they can be detected at the first examination. *Their presence in the sputum is hence one of the
most constant,—if not the most constant—sign of
pulmonary tuberculosis.* Moreover this sign is the
most delicate test for the disease, for different
observers, myself included, have met with cases,
revealed by microscopic .examination, in which the
physical exploration gave an ambiguous result at the
time, while the subsequent course of the disease confirmed the diagnosis. This sign is besides the earliest
objective indication of pulmonary tuberculosis, for
Hiller† has detected the characteristic bacilli in the
blood and scant expectoration of two patients, afflicted
with the initial pulmonary hæmorrhage, while in a
third case of this kind there was not enough sputum
to be examined. Lichtheim has also diagnosed acute
phthisis dating back but a fortnight, by means of the
microscope. Examination of the sputum should, therefore, be resorted to in all doubtful cases.

The bacillus tuberculosis has also been detected by
Lichtheim in the stools in intestinal tuberculosis,
while Rosenstein‡ and Babes§ have found it in the

*Berliner Klin. Wochenschrift, Nos. 7 and 8, 1883.
†Deutsche Med. Wochenschrift, No. 47, 1882.
‡Centralblatt f. d. med. Wissenschaften, Feb. 3rd, 1883.
§Centralblatt, March 3rd, 1883.

urine in tuberculosis of the urinary organs. Finally Fraenkel *has availed himself of the presence of the bacillus tuberculosis as an evidence of the tubercular nature of doubtful laryngeal ulcerations. In some twenty cases he could detect the parasites, at least once in three examinations, on searching for them in the secretion removed with a laryngeal brush.

---

*Berliner Klin. Wocheuschrift, Nos. 3 and 4, 1883.

LECTURE VII.

Glanders.—Typhoid Fever.—Relapsing Fever.—Small-Pox.—Cow-Pox.—
Sheep-Pox.—Measles.—Malaria.— Diphtheria.— Leprosy.—Syphilis.
—The Milk-Epidemic in Aberdeen.

GLANDERS

has recently been added to the list of diseases of known origin. The most decisive researches were made at the laboratory of the German board of health by Loeffler and Schuetz.* In the ulcerated tissues and typical nodules taken from the horse, bacilli were found in limited numbers in and outside of the cells. They resembled the Bacillus Tuberculosis in shape and size, but were readily stained by methyl-blue. They could be cultivated on the surface of solidified serum of the horse and sheep. Their inoculation produced in rabbits and guinea-pigs a fatal disease, beginning with nodular growths, which extended from the spot of inoculation to internal organs. The identity of this affection with genuine glanders was proven by reproducing the disease in its typical form in the animal, which it commonly attacks, viz: the horse. Since this disease

---

* Deutsche Med. Wochenschrift, No. 52, 1882.

can also affect the human being, the—as yet small—
list of human evils traceable to bacterial invasion is
thus increased by one.

A corroboration of these researches has appeared
independently by Israel,* who had for some time previously found the same micro-organism in the pus and
nodules of glanders of the horse. He had also cultivated them on the surface of solidified serum and
obtained with the pure culture an affection in rabbits,
which possessed all the characteristic lesions of glanders. He has had no chance as yet to inoculate
horses. In the pus of closed abscesses in glandered
horses the bacilli were not seen. Almost at the same
time there has also appeared a French publication by
Bouchard, Capiton and Charrin,† who have found micro-organisms in the disease, but who do not give a
sufficient description of their appearance to enable one
to identify them with the bacilli of the Germans. Still
they have cultivated them successfully in broth and
have obtained in sixty-one different rodents a disease
identical with the form in which glanders appears in
them on direct inoculation with the tissues of the
diseased horse.

TYPHOID FEVER.

In this disease various observers (Recklinghausen,
Klein and others) have found colonies of micrococci in
the blood-vessels and in the midst of the tissues. But
this is by no means always the case; quite often these
micro-organisms are not present in the cadaver. Moreover, since they do not differ in appearance from the
colonies of micrococci found in other diseases of the
septic type, there is no good reason why they should

*Berliner Klinische Wochenschrift, No. 11, 1883.
†Bulletin of the Academie de Medicine, No. 51, 1882.

be considered as related to the cause of the disease. Perhaps they represent only a complication.

A well-characterized bacillus, however, has been found in this disease by Eberth.* It is a short, thick rod, of delicate contour, with rounded ends, often with vacuole-like spots in its interior, perhaps spores. He has found it chiefly in the intestinal follicles, but also in the mesenteric glands and the spleen. It stains easily, when the fluid is scraped off the fresh tissue and dried on a cover-glass, but Eberth could not demonstrate it well in stained sections. Hence he used acetic acid as a reagent, whereby he could only detect it in groups, but not, when scattered through the tissue. He found it only in about one half of his cases of typhoid fever, of which he examined twenty-three instances in his first publication. It was present especially during the earlier part of the course of the disease. While its absence in one half of the cases is as yet unexplained, it can hardly be denied that this parasite has some important relation to the disease, since its frequent presence has been confirmed by others, while Eberth, who has sought for it, has never met with it in any other disease. Independently of Eberth, Koch † has discovered the same bacillus, which he illustrates in some photographs. Like Eberth, he found it in only about half of the cases. Since he succeeded in staining it well by using warm solutions, it is not likely that its presence in the negative cases was overlooked. He detected it in the liver, spleen and kidney as well as the intestinal follicles. The same bacilli were seen also by Meyer ‡ (under Friedlander's guidance) in seventeen of twenty-three cases.

---

* Virchow's Archiv. Bd. 81., p. 58, and Bd. 83, p. 486.
† Mittheilungen, &c. p. 45.
‡ Dissertation, 1881. Abstracted in Centralblatt No. 26, 1882.

They were only sought for in the intestinal canal, where they exist in the interior of the swollen patches and in the lymphatic spaces of the external tunics, while they were not found in cadavers dead of other diseases. They have been detected, furthermore, by Coats* and by Cooke,† each in one case. The causal relation of this parasite to the disease can of course not be affirmed until proven by inoculation experiments, however plausible this suspicion may appear.

Klebs‡ has described a different bacillus in typhoid fever. It forms long filaments, up to 0.08 millimeters, but extremely thin (0.2 micromillimeters). These threads increase somewhat in thickness during their growth, then divide into short segments, in which spores appear thereupon. They were detected both in the ulcerated Peyerian patches and in various intestinal organs as well as in the blood-vessels. But since staining methods were not used, their alleged discovery in internal organs must be received with caution, to say the least. In the intestinal lesions they disappear towards the end of the disease. Klebs claims to have cultivated these bacilli in solutions of isinglass and inoculated with them a few different animals. Some of the rabbits were killed thereby in two days and at the autopsy the bacilli were found in the interior of the intestinal follicles—again in unstained sections. Although there was neither any symptom nor any lesion characteristic of typhoid fever in these few animals, Klebs does not hesitate to call his "bacillus typhus" the cause of the disease. Koch—certainly a competent critic—doubts altogether the importance of Klebs' bacilli, because he could find

---

* Brit. Med. Journal, March, 1882.

† Brit. Med. Journal, July, 1882.

‡ Archiv. f. experiment. Pathologie, Bd. XIII.

them only in the necrotic tissue, which offers no resistance to the invasion of any parasites coming from the
intestinal surface, that hot-bed of micro-organisms.
Meyer, likewise, has met with these filaments only in
the necrotic patches open to *post-mortem* invasion.

Tizzoni * has isolated bacteria from drinking water
by filtration, during an epidemic of typhoid fever.
Injected under the skin of animals these gave rise to
the intestinal symptoms of the disease and in the
lesions the same micrococci and delicate mycelia were
found as in the disease of man. It would be unfair
to criticise this work without reading the original, but
the abstract to which I have access does not let it
appear very trustworthy.

A similar want of reliability is apparent in the publication of Brantlecht.† In the urine of typhoid patients
and in drinking water, suspected as the source of
infection, he found a species of bacteria, forming in
the water an iridescent scum on standing in closed
vessels in the warmth. On cultivation in solutions
of gelatine containing phosphate of ammonium, he
obtained whitish flakes consisting of very thin but
long, immovable filaments, which segmented into short
rods and ultimately into granules, perhaps representing
spores. Their growth was quite slow. The injection of
these bacteria under the skin of rabbits produced a slight
rise of temperature, one of 0.5 to 1.5° C. (which means
nothing in the rabbit) lasting less than two days.
But this was followed by emaciation, rarely by diar-
rhoea, leading to the death of the animal in four to
eight weeks. At the autopsy (in sixty-nine cases)
catarrh of the small intestines, swelling of the mesenteric glands and of the spleen was observed. But all

* Abstracted in Revue des Sciences Med., October, 1881, p. 718.
† Virchow's Archiv., Bd. 84, p. 80.

these lesions are not characteristic of typhoid fever in man, while the intestinal ulcerations which Brantlecht did not find, are positive evidence of the disease. Since, hence, neither symptoms nor lesions corresponded to the disease in man, since the fluids were anything but pure cultures and since the parasites were not even looked for in the human tissues, there is really no light thrown upon the cause of the disease by these researches. It may be of interest to add, however, that the bacteria which Brantlecht studied, gradually lost their virulence by continued artificial cultivation and the mild, non-fatal attack, which they then produced gave the animals immunity against a second inoculation. Whatever the disease, which he obtained in rabbits, may have been, the mode of infection, which we suspect on just grounds in typhoid fever, viz: through the intestinal canal, did not succeed with any certainty in that disorder.

Maragliano * has examined the blood of fifteen typhoid fever patients during life—partly from the finger, partly drawn from the spleen. During the height of the fever he found numerous round. granules and to a less extent bacilli, which he compares with those of Klebs and Eberth without distinguishing between the two different kinds.

RELAPSING FEVER

is invariably accompanied by the presence of a parasite in the blood—the *Spirochœte of Obermeier*, who discovered it in 1873. The regular occurrence of this spirillum during the fever has been confirmed by so many different authors in hundreds of cases, that its significance cannot be doubted. Some exceptions have

---

* Centralblatt f. d. Med. Wiss., No. 41, 1882.

also been reported, but there is no evidence that those authors sought for them with sufficient care, certainly not with the aid of staining methods. It is a slender twisted filament about twelve to forty-three micromillimeters long, comparable in shape to a corkscrew, there being some four to ten narrow turns. In the living state it shows usually a lively movement, an eel-like twisting, varying with a rotation around a central axis, as well as telescopic changes in length due to winding and unwinding of the coils. As the blood clots on the slide, the spirilla seek the clear spaces filled with serum (Vandyke Carter*). The parasite seems adhesive and often sticks to blood corpuscles. On the slide, kept moist, it has a tendency to form densely-matted clusters, which are also found at times in the *post-mortem* blood. The parasite has, so far, been found only in the blood and has never been met with in any other disease but recurrent fever. It begins to appear some hours before the first attack of fever, when careful scrutiny will detect a few in each slide. During the febrile paroxysm they increase in number, until they may exceed the number of red-corpuscles, but at the close of the attack, they disappear suddenly. They are not to be found after this time, until a few hours before the characteristic relapses of the diseases. They persist for some hours or days in the blood of the cadaver, provided the patient died during the paroxysm. Both Carter in India and various European authors have reported cases of infection traceable to the performance of an autopsy upon patients.

It is difficult to see the spirilla in the fresh state on account of their delicacy. But in the dried film on the cover-glass they can be better demon-

*Spirillum Fever—1882.

12

strated after clearing with glacial acetic acid or
they may be stained in the usual way with aniline
colors. In the interior of capillaries in sections they
do not take up aniline colors, except brown, and that
but feebly.

Nothing very decisive has been learned in culture
experiments made by different observers. Both Koch
and Carter saw the spirilla elongate considerably and
increase noticeably in thickness on keeping them in
warm glass cells in pure serum or serum diluted with
aqueous humor. They formed dense clusters, gave
indications of segmentation or showed the formation of
bright granules. Yet an unmistakable multiplication
was not observed. They may remain alive for five or
eight days under these circumstances, or even longer
according to other observers, showing occasional, but
sluggish movements. Ultimately they form an aggre-
gation of granules or disappear entirely. Their
gradual appearance could not be watched in blood
taken prior to a relapse, in which no developed spirilla existed as yet. If the germs did pre-exist in the
blood, they could not develop under the circumstances.
Albrecht* took samples of blood at short intervals
before the expected relapse and found successively
free granules, accumulating into groups of six to ten,
elongation of these into the form of chains and transition from such granular chains of zig-zag shape
into perfect spirilla. But he has never seen the continuous development of any one living specimen.
Hence the periodicity of the appearance of the spirilla,
their prompt vanishing at the end of the attack and
the mode of propagation of the parasites are as yet
unsolved problems.

Although the isolation of the spirilla has not yet

*Archiv. f. klin. Medicin, Vol. 29, p. 77.

been accomplished, the disease has been reproduced by inoculation with blood containing the parasites, while the blood of the same patients, taken at times when no spirilla were present, was wholly inactive. Attempts by Obermeier and his various successors have shown the ordinary domestic animals to be insusceptible to the disease, but both Carter and Koch* have succeeded in the monkey.   Carter† inoculated twenty-two monkeys with human blood containing the parasites and obtained infection sixteen times.   In seven of eleven attempts the disease was also transmitted from one animal to another.   Why exceptions occurred was not learned.   Blood taken from the same patients both human and animal during the afebrile period proved harmless.   In the monkey neither the characteristic relapses nor complications occur, the fever, though sometimes fatal, being of shorter duration than in man.   But the nature of the inoculated disease is definitely established by the presence of the spirilla in the blood during the attack.   That the blood containing the spirilla is infectious has furthermore been proven by Motschutkowsky‡ in successful inoculations of human beings.   The disease confers no immunity upon man or monkey.   Both Carter and Koch succeeded in inoculating the same animals twice.

The eruptive fevers of man, so eminently contagious, have not yet been experimentally studied to any satisfactory extent, as far as the nature of the virus is concerned.   In

SMALL–POX

microccoci were discovered by Luginbuehl§ in sec-

*Mittheilungen, etc., p. 166.
†Spirillum Fever, p. 429.
‡Abstr. in Centralblatt f. d. med. Wissensschafter, 1876, No. 11.
§Abstr. in Schmidt's Jahrbuecher, Vol. 166., p. 217.

tions cleared with acetic acid. They formed colonies between the corium and epithelium of the skin, principally in the papules, but also to a less extent between them. More extensive and numerous have been the observations by Weigert.* It was he who principally introduced the staining methods for bacteria, though he did not at that time use the best illumination. He detected microccoci in zooglœa masses in every instance of papules not too far progressed, where they existed at the border of the corium and epidermis. These cocci formed also embolic masses in the blood-vessels of internal organs. Both in the skin and in the viscera each developed colony was surrounded by necrotic tissue, evidently the result of the parasitic action. The micrococci colonies in internal organs in variola are also illustrated by photographs in Koch's " Mittheilungen aus dem kaiserlichen Gesundheitsamte." Micrococci in twos and fours have likewise been seen by Klebs† in the tracheal mucous of small-pox patients, and in the contents of vaccine pustules. No culture experiments have as yet been reported in this disease. It is not improbable, that the micrococci, which constitute the granules in

COW-POX VIRUS

represent the mitigated small-pox parasites. In spite of numerous failures in the hands of a French commission headed by Chauveau and of other experimenters (Klein) we cannot deny, that Ceely and that Babcock did really succeed, though but a few times, in inoculating the heifer with small-pox virus and producing thereby genuine cow-pox, transmissible as

---

*Abstr. in Schmidt's Jahrbuecher, Vol. 166, p. 217.
†Archiv. f. experimentelle Path., Vol. X.

such to the human arm. Evidently the conditions necessary for the transformation of the small-pox poison ·into the mitigated form of cow-pox virus are not yet understood. Perhaps the most light is thrown upon the subject by the recent researches of Voigt,* who found that the virus of the human disease must be passed through several animal generations—the bodies of some six cows in succession—until its virulence is sufficiently reduced to produce in man but the localized form of disease, which suffices for immunity. The hope seems reasonable, that the conditions of mitigation can be better studied, after the active elements have once been isolated.

In the vaccine lymph numerous micrococci are found, according to the testimony of all observers. The same granules have been invariably seen by Pohl-Pincus† in the extirpated papules and pustules produced by vaccination in the calf. They existed both in colonies and scattered throughout the epithelium. In the slight inflammatory reaction caused by a second vaccination of the animal after the lapse of a fortnight, these micrococci could not gain a foothold. Although these parasites have never been separately cultivated it was shown long ago by Chauveau in experiments now classical,‡ that the active principle of the lymph of cow-pox, horse-pox, and sheep-pox consists of granules insoluble in the serum. For when he carefully poured a stratum of water upon a layer of lymph in tiny tubes, he obtained a diffusion of the dissolved material into the water, but this clear solution could not produce pustules like the insoluble residue. On the other hand on diluting the lymph with water there

*Quoted in the " Medical News " Oct. 21st, 1882.

†Wirkung der Vaccination, Abstr. in Centralblatt, No. 25, 1882.

‡Comptes Rendus, 1868.

was no enfeeblement noticeable in its action, as there would be were the active agent in the fluid state. When the lymph was diluted with fifty times as much water, the effect of an inoculation with this mixture became uncertain, but when a pustule did develop it possessed all its typical characteristics. These results can only be interpreted as indicating the corpuscular nature of the active agent. The virus of

SHEEP-POX

has been isolated by Toussaint* in the form of bacilli of the length of three to four micromillimeters. They could be grown in broth in which they showed lively movements, elongated and then divided into two segments of unequal length, in which there appeared one or two spores. The inoculation of sheep gave rise to pustules, which do not seem to have been as well developed, as those produced by the original lymph.

In the urine of patients with

MEASLES

LeBel† has just discovered a "vibrio" about one micromillimeter thick and of variable length, endowed with slow movement and producing spores. The same bacteria were also found in the furfuraceous scales of the skin and were not met with in other diseases. A different observation at least equally reliable is that by Keating,‡ who detected micrococci in the living blood of measles, but only in severe cases. The same microorganism existed in the cutaneous lesions of all pa-

---

* Comptes Rendus, Vol. 92, p. 362.

† Comptes Rendus, No. 1, 1883.

‡ Philadelphia Med. Times, No. 384, 1882.

tients. He does not seem to have made use of staining methods, however.

MALARIAL FEVERS

have proven an encouraging field for etiological researches. The older results of Salisbury and others, who attributed the cause of these disorders to palmelloid growths, have not been confirmed at all by any modern research conducted with more rigorous methods. In 1879 Klebs and Tommasi-Crudeli * announced the discovery of a "bacillus malariæ," the spores of which were obtained from the soil and the air of malarial districts. These spores, slightly less than a micromillimeter in size grew into long threads, subsequently segmenting, in solutions of gelatine and in miniature mud-swamps. Their growth required the presence of oxygen. Their injection into the bodies of rabbits produced a fever lasting several days, with some diurnal fluctuations of the temperature. These animals, when killed, showed considerable enlargement of the spleen and the presence of black pigment in that organ and in the blood. In the blood, the spleen and the marrow of the bones, the bacilli were found in the form of threads 0.06 to 0.084 millimeters long and 0.6 micromillimeters wide. Now this may be malaria, but since we do not know in what form the disease does appear in rabbits, the experiments furnish really no convincing proof. Sternberg † on repeating them with bacilli obtained from the mud at New Orleans, could not confirm these results, but that is not saying, that he refuted them, as he himself admits, for he may not have had the same micro-organism. Marchiafava and Cuboni ‡ have subsequently detected

---

* Archiv. f. experimentelle Path., Vol. 11.

† National Board of Health, Supplement No. 14, July, 1881.

‡ Archiv. f. experimentelle Path., Bd. 13.

granules in the blood of malarial patients, which they tried to identify with the spores of Klebs and Tommasi-Crudeli. They also saw a few bacilli. They injected the blood óf human patients into the veins of dogs and obtained a somewhat intermittent fever. Marchand * published later some casual observations, made some years previously on a malarial patient, in whose blood he found granules and a few movable rods with spore-like swellings at the ends corresponding to Klebs' description, but only during the paroxysm. Ziehl † detected similar bacilli, few in number, in the blood of three fever patients. After the cure of two of these by quinine the micro-organisms disappeared. Of twenty-five other non-malarial individuals examined in this respect, only one showed the presence of these bacilli in the blood. It was a case of diabetes, possibly of malarial origin, for it was cured by quinine, whereupon the bacilli disappeared. Finally Ceci ‡ has cultivated the spores of malarial earth (under Klebs' guidance) in artificial swamps, and in solutions of gelatine, and claims that the power of these bacilli, to produce an intermittent fever in rabbits, diminishes on continued artificial cultivation. But I can find no evidence at all in his article, that the bacteria cultivated really produced anything like a malarial affection. Hence however plausible the doctrine of the "Bacillus Malariæ" may sound, the experimental supports furnished by the school of Klebs are as yet insufficient and not convincing.

An entirely different micro-organism Laveran§ claims to have detected in the blood of some forty out of

---

* Virchow's Archiv., Band 88, p. 104.
†Deutsche Med. Wochenschrift, Nov. 25, 1882.
‡Archiv. f. experimentelle Path., Vols. 15 and 16.
§Comptes Rendus, Vol. 93, No. 17.

sixty malarial patients and never in other diseases.
He describes three forms, viz.: 1. Oval corpuscles,
slightly larger than red blood-disks drawn out at both
ends and pigmented in the center. 2. Spherical corpuscles about six micromillimeters in size with numerous pigment granules and, when in motion, extending
out long delicate processes from the periphery. 3.
Granulated spherical motionless globules about 0.01
millimeters in size, apt to change into irregular plates.
He considers these three fanciful forms but different
phases in the development of an animal parasite. But
as he has neither cultivated nor isolated the alleged
parasite and has not even shown, that it is not an
altered blood-corpuscle, no further conclusions of
course can be drawn from his researches. The same
suspense of judgment must be maintained with reference to the statements of Richard,* who claims to
have made similar observations on the existence of
this parasitic animal in the malarial blood.

DIPHTHERIA.

In the pseudo-membranes of 'this disease bacteria of
different kinds occur in large numbers. This, indeed,
might be expected in the case of dead tissues, kept
warm and moist and exposed to the invasion of the
numerous micro-organisms abounding on mucous surfaces. The most constant bacteria met with are
micrococci partly in zoogloea masses of a yellowish
hue. They were first described by Oertel (1868) and
their presence has been confirmed since by many
observers. A very full description is given of them
by Wood and Formad.† They are of various sizes
and are distributed throughout the false membranes,

*Comptes Rendus, Vol. 24, p. 49.
†National Board of Health Bulletin, Supplement No. 17, Jan., 1882.

being partly between, partly in the interior of the remnants of cells. Wood and Formad speak of them as round granules, while Oertel in his late publication* describes them as slender rods 1 by 0.3 micromillimeters and larger ones 4.2 by 1.1 micromillimeters, joined in pairs and in chains, also in zoogloea form. *There is as yet, however, no proof, that these micrococci are the cause of the disease.* Their presence in the exposed *dead* tissue is no evidence, for the membrane represents but the necrotic mucous lining. Indeed, when the healthy mucous membrane of the mouth or trachea is destroyed by caustics, for instance ammonia, the eschar into which it is converted—really a pseudo-membrane—contains the same micrococci, as are found in true diphtheria, as Wood and Formad have learned. Moreover in the scrapings of the healthy tongue the same micrococci can be seen. Of more significance is the detection of the same—or similar—micrococci in the blood of the living patient during severe attacks. But since these parasites were found only in the more severe cases and not in all instances of the disease, were seen also in the blood of other septic disorders, and since no cultures have been made with the fresh blood, there is not yet enough evidence for any decision. In the internal organs bacteria are not found with any regularity in diphtheria. Oertel in Ziemssen's Cyclopædia states, that he has usually met with micrococci in the kidneys in this disease. Eberth, Gaucher and Litten have each seen one instance of bacterial presence in the inflamed kidney in diphtheria, but in other cases, more numerous, they have not been detected by competent investigators. In the heart, spleen and liver bacterial colonies have

---

*Vortraege in Aerztlichen Verein zu Muenchen, Zur Ætiologie der Infections krankheiten, 1881, p. 225.

been, but not invariably found. Their arrangement resembled strikingly the lesions of pyæmia. Hence the occasional presence of bacteria in the viscera presents probably but an accidental complication of diphtheria.

Many of the attempts at inoculation of animals with diphtherial material throw no light whatever upon the nature of this disease. For quite often the membranes were put under the skin of animals, where they started a destructive inflammation, resembling hospital gangrene. Now this is not at all diphtheria, as we see it clinically. It is true the Germans speak of "diphtheria of wounds," but it is yet to be proven, that this process is identical as to its cause with the diphtheria of mucous membranes. Clinically we speak of diphtheria only, when there occurs a *spreading destruction of a mucous membrane, converting it into a pseudomembrane.* This alone is the essence of the disease, every thing else is secondary. Such a destruction of the epithelial and often also of the deeper layers of a mucous lining appears as a false membrane, no matter whether it be caused by mechanical or chemical influences or by the specific diphtherial virus, *but in the latter case only will the process extend,* while chemical injuries give rise to the same appearance, limited, however, to the spot originally involved. Hence the application of caustics and of heat to mucous surfaces causes the same pseudo-membranes, which neither the naked eye nor the microscope can distinguish from the genuine diphtherial products. But these false membranes do not increase beyond their original size. In order to recognize the diphtheritic virus, we must therefore apply it to mucous membranes as a test. This has been done, but such an inoculation does not always take effect.

Trendelenburg succeeded but eleven times in fifty-two trials, on placing human pseudo-membranes into the trachea of rabbits and pigeons. Wood and Formad had but two successes in thirty-six inoculations with material taken from mild cases of the disease, while with more virulent membranes from epidemic cases five infections occurred in ten attempts. Twice they also transferred the membrane from one animal to another. Now this is sufficient to prove the inoculability of the disease. As regards the explanation of the failures, we must take into account the varying susceptibility of animals, for the rabbit is not known to take diphtheria spontaneously, as well as our ignorance as regards the diphtherial virus and whether it is not "crowded out" of the false membranes by other bacteria. The inoculability of the disease does not prove bacteria to be the cause, however likely this may be. As regards culture experiments I can only find a record of them in the numerous publications by Letzerich and the report by Wood and Formad. The former author, working with the most defective methods and jumping at conclusions on the basis of few and most inadequate experiments, cannot demand any belief for his assertions. Such productions can only bring the germ-theory into discredit. The American observers, however, have cultivated micrococci from the diphtherial membranes by methods perfectly reliable,—only the material from which they took their germs, the membranes, contained of course any number of accidental germs. Hence there is no proof positive, that the crop which they did get, represented the parasites of diphtheria. Moreover they cultivated apparently the same micrococci from scrapings of the tongue. They found that these micrococci could not grow indefinitely in a broth of rabbit, but that the vegetation

became feebler in each successive transfer to a fresh
soil. The micrococci of tongue scrapings showed the
feeblest power of multiplication, while the bacteria
from the membranes of severe cases of diphtheria
could be cultivated through some eight or nine successive generations. As they claim, other bacteria did
not enter their flasks. This limitation of the power of
reproduction is so entirely different from what has
been observed in other bacteria, that it .requires confirmation and further study before it can be accepted
as proven. All other bacteria, that have been studied,
retain their unlimited power of reproduction on transfer to a fresh soil, if this soil is at all adequate for
their vegetation.

The inoculation of eight rabbits in the trachea with
the micrococci cultivated by Wood and Formad, gave a
wholly negative result, while in thirteen other instances
injection into the muscles showed likewise, that these
bacteria could not cause anything like diphtheria. How
the authors can hence identify these micrococci with
the cause of diphtheria, I cannot understand. They
also believe to have isolated the micrococci in another
manner, viz: by filtration of the urine of diphtherial
patients and inoculation with the filter-paper. But
they do not state, what kinds of bacteria the urine
contained, relying on the worthless statements by
Letzerich, that there are only micrococci present, and
with the paper thus employed they produced *pyæmia*
in two rabbits and nothing at all in two others.
While these researches cannot therefore prove the
bacterial origin of diphtheria, this presumption is not
disproven by the experiments of Satterthwaite and
Curtis.* For the latter observers, who claim, that
they can obtain results identical with those produced

* Report to the New York Board of Health, 1877. I did not have

by pseudo-membranes, by the inoculation with putrid
fluids, did not at all produce diphtheria in animals,
but only some form of blood-poisoning or local inflammation and destructive phlegmons. They injected under
the skin or into the muscles and hence did not
search for the diphtherial virus by any adequate test.

Klebs,* who has by this time discovered the germs
of almost every disease, has found in the diphtherial
membranes the "micrococcus diphthericus" in the
form of "micrococci balls" (zoogloea?), which become
transformed into minute rods and ultimately into delicate mycelium growing in the tissues. Like all of
Klebs' bacteria, these forms were cultivated in solutions of isinglass. Their injection produced blood-
poisoning without any characteristic appearances of
diphtheria.

Some ten years ago Eberth produced—what he
called—diphtheria of the cornea, by inoculation with
membranes, later on also with pyæmic pus. The
same result was then obtained by Dolschenkow,† Leber
and others with common putrid material and also with
mould-fungi. But this is simply a necrosis of the
cornea due to bacterial invasion and bears no resemblance whatever to true diphtheria.

Entirely different are the observations of Talamon.‡
In the false membranes examined fresh he found an
organism, which could be regarded as a higher fungus.
He did not examine any sections of human tissues
and hence cannot state anything about its occurrence
anywhere, except in the membranes. In some of the
viscera, however, of the inoculated animals the same

---

the original, but know it from the quotation by Wood and Formad
(*loc. cit.*) and Jacobi "On Diphtheria."

    * Archiv. f. experimentelle Pathologie, Vol. IV.

    †Vide Centralblatt, 1873.

    ‡Progres Medical, Feb. 17 and June 25, 1881.

fungus was found. No staining methods were used
and hence no reliable details were brought forth.
With the membranes culture solutions were infected,
what kind, and in what, arrangement is not stated.
As the result he observed the development of a continuous mycelium some two to five micromillimeters
thick, and partitioned off by transverse septa. The
places of bifurcation resembled the branches of a
tuning-fork or lyre. In other less favorable cases
there were only thick rods arranged like crutches,
some fifteen to forty micromillimeters long. The
spores were oval, three to five micromillimeters in
size and often grouped in zoogloea masses. There
were also "conidia" rectangular in shape, several times
as large as the spores, arranged frequently in chains.
All these forms were of gigantic dimensions, when
compared with bacteria. Why, hence, did they escape
the observation of other investigators? I can only
find a record of some observations by Nix,* who saw
similar fungi in diphtherial membranes in Norway
without knowing of Talamon's work.

Talamon inoculated a variety of animals with his
cultures. Various rabbits, guinea-pigs, frogs and
chickens died, containing these fungi in their tissues.
But in none of these instances were there any appearances of diphtheria. In four pigeons, however, he
obtained genuine pseudo-membranes in the mouth,
which contained the fungi. In some kittens, dead of
spontaneous diphtheria, acquired in the laboratory, the
same micro-organisms were detected in the membranes
and viscera. Talamon's statements are so startling, that
it is best to wait for further confirmation, or at least
for more precise details, than he has published so far.

---

* Abstr. in Jahresbericht ueber die Leistungen in der Med., 1881,
Bd. I, Abth. II, p. 389.

LEPROSY.

As far as mere observation can prove, this affection is one of bacterial origin. More cautiously speaking, it can be stated, that characteristic bacilli are invariably found in leprous growths, but their importance has not yet been established absolutely, as it only can be by isolation and inoculation. They were discovered by Hansen * and further studied by Neisser,† Cornil, and by Koebner.‡ They have been found in every case of leprosy examined by these authors and several others.§ The "bacillus lepræ" is a very delicate rod, about one half the length of a red blood disc and one fourth as wide as long, tapering at the ends. The rod may be thickened by several nodosities — the spores. It is found scattered or in interlaced groups, or in articulated chains, mainly in the 'interior of the cells and only in the leprous infiltrations of the tissues, not in healthy parts. The so-called lepra-cells or globi constitute the remnants of degenerated animal cells, choked with large clusters of bacilli. The parasites exist in all the leprous tissues, but have not been found in the blood except by Koebner (and by Gaucher in a rather doubtful manner). In the skin the bacilli appear as separate short rods, but in internal organs Cornil‖ describes them as long unsegmented filaments. The bacilli, which have some active motion, while alive, can be recognized only with difficulty in the fresh specimen, better after the application of

---

* Norwegian publication in 1873, and Virchow's Archiv., 1880, Bd. 79, I.

† Virchow's Archiv., Bd. 85, p. 514.

‡ Virchow's Archiv., Bd. 88, p. 282.

§ Dr. Schmidt of New Orleans claims to have been unable to demonstrate them, but his slides, which I have seen, were stained imperfectly and diffusely and were not examined with a proper condenser.

‖ Bull. of the Paris Academie de Med., No. 3, 1881.

dilute potash solution (1 in 12). In sections of hardened tissues they stain well with fuchsin, less perfectly with violet. Koebner recommends drying the tissues before they are hardened in alcohol. Coverglass films of fluid can be stained readily, but the bacilli are not visible until the specimen has been partly decolorized in alcohol.

The bacilli have been cultivated in serum on hollow slides by Neisser, and lately on the surface of bloodserum and gelatine mixtures by Hansen.* Their growth is rather slow, and requires a high temperature. In meat-broth Hansen could not get them to vegetate. Their spores appear at first as nodular thickenings of the filaments; later on they may be set free. The decisive experiment of inoculating animals with isolated bacilli has not yet succeeded, though attempted by Neisser, Koebner and Hansen,—probably because the domestic animals possess an immunity against the disease. Even in a monkey Koebner has failed to obtain any infection by means of transplanted nodules.

Since it is believed in the East, that the disease exists amongst fishes, Koebner has also tried some of these animals, but likewise with no success. Leprosy can hence not yet be ranged amongst the diseases of proven bacterial origin.

It is of interest to note, that in three diseases, classed by pathologists as "infectious granulation tumors," viz: tuberculosis, glanders and leprosy, the invariable presence of bacilli has been demonstrated. In the fourth member of that group, viz:

SYPHILIS,

our knowledge is as yet imperfect. Klebs † has culti-

* Virchow's Archiv., Bd. 90, p. 542.
† Archiv. f. experimentelle Path., Vol. X.

13

vated in egg albumen granules and short twisted rods
on placing bits of an excised chancre into it. This
micro-organism he termed "Helicomonas." He could
not demonstrate its presence, however, in any unopened lesion. Inoculation experiments with the original syphilitic products succeeded only in the monkey,
not in other animals, and then but occasionally. In
one case, however, he had an undoubted success, as
his description indicates to any one familiar with the
disease. But on inoculating with the cultivated heli-
comonads, the experiments were all of the most ambiguous kind. In view of the unreliability of Klebs'
culture experiments, there is hence no conclusion to
be drawn from this research.

Subsequently Aufrecht* described large oval micrococci in the interior of specific condylomata. Essentially the same things have been seen by Birch-
Hirschfeld.† He spoke in his first communication of
short rods, but corrected himself afterwards and now
recognizes only oval micrococci, mostly in pairs and
sometimes in the form of chains. They are readily
shown by staining with fuchsin. He claims to have
found them invariably in more than twelve gummatous
tumors of internal organs, in three excised specific
warts, in an extirpated chancre and in a syphilitic
papule. They were not seen in the blood.

Different again is the description by Morrison,‡ of
what he found in the secretions of fifteen different
syphilitic lesions. Some of these were papules not
ulcerated, and hence not exposed to the air. Moreover, sections were made from one chancre and two
papules. The sections and dried cover-glass films

---

*Centralblatt f. d. med. Wissenschaften, No. 13, 1881.

†Centralblatt, Nos. 33 and 44, 1882.

‡Maryland Med. Journal, Jan. 1st, 1883.

were put into acetic acid, then transferred to alcohol and dried and thereupon stained with methyl-blue or with fuchsin and decolorized in dilute nitric acid (1 in 6). In all specimens he found small rods (quite thick in his drawing), usually in groups. In the pus of soft chancres he found longer, but very thin bacilli, different from those in genuine syphilis.

Of culture experiment and inoculation I can find a record only in the publication of Martineau and Hamonic,* which appeals to the imagination rather than to criticism. Pasteur's solution of tartrate of ammonium, in which no one has as yet succeeded in growing pathogenic bacteria, was infected with a piece from an excised chancre. In twenty-two hours it swarmed with "bacteridia." These were injected into a pig, their progeny was found in the blood on the next day, and a month later ｉthere appeared a papulo-squamous eruption and falling out of the bristles. A somewhat similar result, following the inoculation with a piece of the original chancre, is to prove, that this disease of the pig is really syphilis. Fresh cultures made from the bacteria in the blood of these infected animals did not prove infectious to other animals. So much for the etiology of syphilis from that source!

THE MILK-FEVER EPIDEMIC IN ABERDEEN

was an instance of a hitherto unknown affection, occurring suddenly in an epidemic form, and traceable to the accidental diffusion of the bacteria producing it. The disease, described by I. Cossar Ewart,† attacked within a short time some three hundred people. It began with a chill followed by high fever, often with

---

*Comptes Rendus, No. 10, Vol. 95.

†Brit. Med. Journal, Nov. 4, 1882.

delirium, while the characteristic symptom was a swelling of the deep cervical glands. In twenty-four to forty-eight hours it had usually terminated, leaving behind considerable exhaustion. Sometimes relapses were observed involving other lymphatic glands. The cause of the epidemic was traced to the use of milk coming from one dairy. This milk had been watered. In the diluted milk and in the cistern from which the water was taken, a bacillus resembling the bacillus anthracis was detected. In one of the patients the swollen glands suppurated and in the pus the same bacilli were found. Rats inoculated with the parasites died in eighteen to twenty-four hours. The bacilli were found vegetating in the tissues. But the description does not indicate, whether the experimental disease in the rats presented the same symptoms and lesions as the human affection. Hence the evidence as to the bacterial origin of the epidemic is not conclusive, though very suggestive.

LECTURE VIII.

Local Diseases. — Inflammations. — Gonorrhœa and Gonorrhœal Conjunctivitis. — Trachoma. — Croupous Pneumonia. — Endocarditis.— Inflammations of Diathetic Origin.—Sympathetic Ophthalmia.— Whooping-Cough.—Rhinoscleroma.—Pterygium.—Carious Teeth.— The Poison of Rhus Toxicodendron.—The Importance and Future of the Germ-Theory.—Parasitic Mould-Fungi.—Actinomycosis.

Most of the diseases, the ætiology of which we have thus far reviewed, are classified in the books as constitutional disorders. The revelations of the germ-theory, however, point out that the distinction between constitutional and local diseases can no longer be strictly maintained in the former sense. Of course a disease strictly localized and not affecting the rest of the system, is a local disorder, no matter from what point of view we regard it. But some of the affections, which have been considered of constitutional significance, for instance typhoid fever, erysipelas and—as we shall see presently — croupous pneumonia, amount really to a localization of the parasite in some part, with only secondary involvement of the system at large, due probably to the absorption of morbid products, be they generated by the bacteria or set free by the

activity of the diseased tissues. Strictly constitutional are only those affections, in which the virus
exists in the blood throughout the entire body, for
instance anthrax and septicæmia. At any rate the line
between the two classes of diseases cannot be drawn
sharply, because in some local affections the active
agent enters the blood secondarily, to be deposited
somewhere else. However, these are all merely suggestions. Our knowledge is yet too imperfect to discuss the subject much on the basis of facts.

The most frequent of all local disorders—inflammation—has been traced to parasitic influence in some
few instances. We have discussed previously, that the
suppurative inflammation of wounds and of abscesses
is generally produced by the micrococci described by
Ogston. It must be remembered, however, that suppurative inflammation is a reaction of the tissues,
which can be induced by a sufficient irritation of
chemical nature, as well as by the presence of certain
bacteria, only the former cause is not so common.
Undoubtedly various different species of bacteria can
produce suppurative reaction of the tissues. Thus,
besides the micrococcus of Ogston, we have learned that
the pyæmia 'micrococcus of Koch and the "vibrio" of
Pasteur, the micrococcus of progressive gangrene (Koch)
all start suppuration. As we shall further see, a similar result follows the invasion of the tissues by a
higher fungus, the actinomyces. Probably other
parasitic causes of suppuration may yet be discovered.
In some instances of parasitic disease the occurrence
of suppuration is probably a secondary matter, due to
the subsequent entrance of other germs. Thus tuberculosis in the viscera does not always result in the
formation of pus, in some organs like the brain—
never, while in localities exposed to the air, as the

lungs, the growth of the bacillus tuberculosis is complicated by some other influence causing suppuration.

A special form of suppurative inflammation, which has always been recognized as due to a specific virus, viz:

GONORRHŒA,

has been traced definitely to the invasion by a distinct and well-characterized parasite. Neisser* described as the "gonococcus" a large round granule, mostly in pairs (forming thus a characteristic biscuit-shaped diplococcus) and often in zoogloea colonies of ten to twenty or more. It exists partly free, partly on the surface of the pus cells, less often the epithelial cells. He found it only in the pus of gonorrhœa (thirty-five cases in the male and two in the female), and of the eye-disease due to gonorrhœal infection, viz.: blennorrhœal conjunctivitis, and never in purulent fluids of other origin. Neisser's statements have since been confirmed by Leistikow† and by Sternberg with reference to gonorrhœa, and by Hirschberg and Krause‡ and by Haab§ with reference to the contagious inflammation of the conjunctiva. But it must be added Hirschberg and Krause have also seen similar microorganisms, though less in number, in the pus of simple purulent conjunctivitis.

The gonococci have been cultivated by Leistikow and by Krause‖ on the surface of solidified bloodserum, on which they form a thin moist scum growing very slowly. A singular observation was made with reference to the temperature. The first crop,

---

*Centralblatt, No. 28, 1879.
†Charite Annalen, Berlin. 1882. Over two hundred cases.
‡Centralblatt f. Augenheilkunde, Feb. and Sept., 1881.
§Centralblatt f. Augenheilkunde, Sept. 1881.
‖Centralblatt f. Augenheilkunde, May, 1882.

obtained by infecting the soil with the specific pus, could not be cultivated except by exposure to a high temperature. But when a pure culture was once started, its growth did not cease at the ordinary temperature of the room. The virulence of these pure cultures, however, could not be proven, since none of the accessible animals could be infected with gonorrhœa or purulent conjunctivitis by means of either the original pus or the isolated parasites. The inoculation of the cultivated gonococci into the conjunctiva or under the skin of animals, proved harmless. No animal has yet been found susceptible to human gonorrhœa.

A positive result, however, was obtained by Bokai,* on injecting the cultivated gonococci into the urethræ of some medical students. In three cases out of six a genuine gonorrhœa resulted. But not sufficient details are stated to render the observations absolutely convincing. A similar experiment without the least flaw, has been successfully conducted by Bockhart.† The micrococci had been cultivated upon the surface of a gelatinous solution of meat extract and peptone. Of the fourth generation a small quantity was injected with due precautions into the healthy urethra of a bedridden demented patient, whose death was expected within a short time. Inside of three days there began a typical gonorrhœa, which lasted until the death of the patient on the tenth day. In the pus the characteristic cocci were found. At the autopsy the micrococci were seen in stained sections between the epithelial cells of the urethral mucous membrane, never in the epithelial cells, but frequently in the interior of pus cells, especially in the nuclei. They had veg-

---

*Allgemeine Med. Centralzeitung, 1880, No. 74.
†Abstracted in Centrablatt f. Chirurgie, No. 9, 1883.

etated in the lymphatic spaces of the submucous tissue, plugging the whole caliber of some of the lymph vessels. Although but one experiment was made by Bockhart, the faultless methods employed, entitle it to full credit. Such a positive observation cannot be overthrown by the failure of another author in the same direction. Sternberg,* confirming Neisser as regards the invariable presence of the characteristic micro-organisms in gonorrhœal pus, has cultivated these bacteria in rabbit broth and placed pellets of cotton saturated with the culture fluids into the urethra of five men (twice in one case) with wholly negative results. Since he has certainly worked with sufficient care, I can think of but two suggestions which might explain his failures. His cultures had all been long continued, the thirteenth and even thirtieth generations being employed. Now we cannot foretell, whether the micrococci retain their virulence forever in culture fluids, hence it would be preferable to test the first or second generation obtained from the original source. Moreover, it is very difficult, if possible, to guarantee, that in the course of thirteen to thirty successive cultivations in fluids, there has not been an entrance of foreign germs, perhaps not distinguishable by the microscope from the bacteria under observation. On the other hand with the use of fluids for cultivating purposes everything depends on the purity of the first material. Sternberg states, that the micrococci which he cultivated from gonorrhœal pus, could transform urea into carbonate of ammonia, were in fact identical with the " micrococcus ureæ." In view of Bockhart's positive result, is it not reasonable to suspect, that Sternberg had the accident of starting his culture with pus containing both the gonococci

*Medical News, Jan. 20th and 27th, 1883.

and the "micrococci ureæ" and that the latter survived alone!

In connection with the origin of purulent conjunctivitis a very important experiment by Sattler* should
be mentioned. The question has often been raised,
whether the purulent ophthalmia of the new-born
child can have any other cause, but the existence of
a specific vaginitis of the mother. In order to decide
this point Sattler put into the eye of a babe six days
old the normal lochial discharge of a perfectly healthy
mother, producing thereby a mild purulent conjunctivitis. The lochial secretion contained a large variety
of bacteria, but not enough of the Gonococci to be
certain of their presence. But in the conjunctival pus
the characteristic micrococci were found in abundance.
In spite of its interest this one experiment does not
seem to me a sufficient basis for further conclusion.

Conjunctival blenorrhœa is not rarely followed by

TRACHOMA.

More commonly, however, this disease begins as
such. In the granulations, characteristic of this
morbid process, Sattler † found invariably a coccus,
slightly smaller than the gonococcus, either single or
in pairs or small groups with an interspace between
the separate granules, but never in zooglœa masses.
It was seen principally on the surface of the—apparently free—nuclei, filling the trachomatous granulations. But it extended also into the depth by
vegetation in the lymph spaces, which were partly
obliterated in long-standing cases. In the pus of the

---

*Bericht der Heidelberger Ophthalmologischen Gesellschaft, 1882,
p. 54.

†Bericht der Heidelberger Ophthalmologischen Gesellschaft, 1881
and 1882.

conjunctival sac the micrococci were not always
present. Sattler has cultivated these parasites both in
fluids on microscopic slides and on the surface of a
gelatine-serum mixture. On the latter soil the culture
appears as a delicate dust growing very slowly. The
third generation of these cultivated micrococci was put
with some friction into a healthy human conjunctival
sac, producing thereby a typical, but mild, trachoma.
The case was observed during several weeks, and then
the diseased portion removed by excision. Previously
Sattler had also obtained the same result by the inoculation with the characteristic micrococci cultivated in
a fluid soil. No success, however, was had on inoculating animals. That the disease, thus produced, was
really characteristic trachoma was guaranteed both by
competent clinical observation, and by the inability to
obtain the specific disease by placing putrid refuse
and cultures of other bacteria on the human conjunctiva. In these experiments Sattler of course took the
precaution to attempt inoculation only, when the
corneal epithelium was' intact. For through an
abrasion of the latter a dangerous suppurative inflammation might have been started by the putrefaction-
bacteria.

Of non-suppurative inflammations very few have as
yet been traced to bacterial invasion. Perhaps the
best known instance is

CROUPOUS PNEUMONIA.

In eight successive cases of this disease Friedlaen-
der* found invariably an oval micrococcus, about one
micromillimeter long and two-thirds as wide, often
joined in pairs. If could be seen in stained sections

*Virchow's Archiv, Vol. 87, p. 319.

in the exsudate filling the alveoli, but its principal
site was in the interior of the lymphatic vessels.
Indeed it gave the latter the appearance of brilliant
cords in sections simply cleared with acetic acid.*
The significance of these micro-organisms, however,
must remain undecided, until inoculation experiments
succeed. Griffini and Cambria have also investigated
the ætiology of pneumonia, finding a bacillus in the
blood and sputa. But in the short abstract † accessible to me, I can find no evidence, that they have
proven anything at all—either in favor of or against
the bacterial origin.

Our knowledge as regards other non-suppurative
inflammations is as yet very meagre. In fact I cannot
point to another clinical instance of a non-suppurative
inflammatory process, definitely traced to the influence
of bacteria, except some secondary complications during
infectious diseases, of which the most common is

ENDOCARDITIS.

This affection, so frequent in the course of pyæmia,
presents always the occurrence of bacteria in the
inflamed tissue and in the fibrinous concretions on its
surface. Koester‡ has traced the parasitic invasion of
the cardiac valves to embolic plugs of bacteria in the
smaller blood-vessels. He suggests, that the movements of the valves during the play of the heart favor
the arrest and deposition in this region of any foreign
particles existing in the blood.——While numerous
pathologists have seen and described the occurrence of
parasites in the pyæmic form of endocarditis I can find

---

*Evidently the same micro-organisms are figured by Koch in a
photograph. Mittheilungen, etc., p. 46.

†Medical News, Dec. 23rd, 1882.

‡Virchow's Archiv. Vol. 72, p. 257.

no further details reported except the statement, that
they are usually micrococci.——In other forms of endocarditis not of pyæmic orign, bacteria have also, but
not invariably, been seen. Klebs insists especially on
the presence of micrococci (or monads, as he calls
them) in the rheumatic heart affections, thus leading
to the inference, that rheumatism is also a parasitic
disease.

In various inflammations, formerly attributed to a
"diathesis" we have now reason to think, that they
originate through the deposition of parasites, existing
in the circulation and that these bacteria develop mainly
in those tissues, where they find the best conditions
for their vegetation. That such a deposition of
circulating parasites can occur I can illustrate by
two examples. When Arloing, Cornevin and Thomas
injected the bacilli of symptomatic charbon into the veins
of cattle, the parasites could not develop to any extent
and the animals did not suffer much. But whenever
an extravasation of blood occurred in the muscles
through an injury, the bacilli found the necessary
conditions for their vegetation in the tissues and produced their usual disastrous effects. Another illustration,
even more to the point, has been furnished by Schueller. In healthy rabbits the contusion of a joint gave
rise to but a temporary irritation. But on injecting
tubercular material into the veins, the circulating virus
was deposited in the injured joints and there resulted
a chronic tubercular inflammation of the joint. Evidently the injury rendered those tissues a favorable
soil for the growth of the bacilli.

A tissue in which inflammations of diathetic origin
are quite commonly seen is the cornea. But on
account of the scarcity of human material no demon-
strations of the presence of bacteria have yet been

furnished. Clinically we can observe a primary suppurative inflammation of the cornea, in which micrococci have been seen by Leber. Since similar forms
have been obtained by inoculations on animals, there
can be little doubt, that this at least is a parasitic
keratitis. Probably the parasites always enter in this
form through some abrasion of the epithelium. But
we know also of several other clinical forms of corneal
disease, which must be regarded as manifestations of
a diathesis or of the existence of some infectious virus
in the body. There is thus a scrofulous, a syphilitic, a
variolous, probably also a malarial keratitis. But I
must repeat, however suggestive the topic is, it has
not yet been worked up.

In the so-much dreaded sympathetic forms of eye
disease the infectious virus, probably their cause, reaches
the second eye, not through the circulation, but by creep-
ing up through the interspaces or between the sheaths
of one optic nerve to the chiasm and thence descending
along the other optic nerve. Such at least is a just
inference from the researches of Knies* and of Leber,†
but the positive demonstration is yet wanting.

Of non-inflammatory diseases I may refer briefly to ·

WHOOPING-COUGH,

in which Burger‡ has regularly found short bacilli
in the sputum on staining films of it. He has not
met with these forms in the expectoration of other
diseases. But of course the mere detection is not
sufficient to demonstrate their importance. The older
fanciful statements by Letzerich as regards the causation of this disease by fungi have not been corroborated and are now discredited by everybody.

---

*Archives of Ophthalmology, Vol. 9, p. 125.
†Archiv. f. Ophthalmologie, Bd. 27, H. I, p. 325.
‡Berliner Klinische Wochenschrift, No. 1, 1883.

RHINOSCLEROMA,

a rare form of progressive induration of the tissues
has been examined by Frisch* in twelve specimens,
partly fresh, partly hardened. In all of these he
found very short bacilli partly between, but mainly in
the interior of the large swollen cells characteristic
of the disease. The bacteria were cultivated on the
surface of gelatine mixtures, but their inoculation did
not succeed in animals. In a case of

PTERYGIUM

Poncet† has detected an extensive colony of bacteria
under the head of the triangular growth, between it
and the corneal tissue. He gives no description of
them, but his drawing makes them appear as micrococci. Their relation to the growth was such that
they must have preceded its development. However
incomplete this observation is, it is certainly suggestive in pointing out the role of bacteria in a disease,
where they never were suspected.

Such hints as this one render it desirable to search
for bacteria in all growths and tumors characterized
by progressiveness. But no reliable observation has
as yet been reported.

CARIOUS TEETH

have been known to harbor bacteria ever since, and
even prior to the researches of Leber and Rottenstein
in 1867. These authors found that the concretions on
teeth—the so-called tartar — contained besides the
earthy salt, the remnants of the leptothrix buccalis,
the articulated filaments found in every human mouth.

---

*Wiener Med. Wochenschrift, 1882, No. 32.
†Archives d' Ophthalmologie, Dec., 1880.

The same micro-organisms penetrate into the tissues of the decaying teeth. But it would be hazardous to say that they cause the decay, seeing that the decayed portion represents practically dead refuse exposed to bacterial invasion. Of more significance are the recent observations by Miller,* who saw the dentine canals in stained sections filled with micro-organisms. Besides the leptothrix there were large bacilli and micrococci. The invasion extended just beyond the border of the carious portion. Still Miller does not claim that the parasites are the only cause of the decay, but seeks the primary impulse rather than in the action of acids.

Finally, as the last example of bacterial agency, and one which seems rather surprising, I may refer to the effect of the

POISON IVY (RHUS TOXICODENDRON)

upon the human body. In the minute vesicles, forming part of the eruption caused by handling this plant, Burrill † has repeatedly seen numerous granules, closely resembling micrococci. The same granules were found in the natural juice of the poison-ivy leaves, and it was further determined that the diluted juice can provoke the irritation of the skin. There are, however, no proofs presented in the paper, that these granules were really micrococci, which question either staining or cultivating methods would have decided. The most convincing observation, which Burrill presents, is the successful infection of a fresh part of the skin with the exudation of the inflamed spot. The array of facts thus far presented, furnishes a

* Archiv f. experimentelle Pathologie, Bd. 16, p. 291.
† American Microscopical Journal, Oct., 1882.

broad basis for a future germ-theory. No matter, whether further research will show, that many more, or—be it few other contagious diseases, are due to the agency of bacteria, the proof *is* absolute, that the invasion by these micro-organisms is the cause of anthrax, chicken cholera, the various forms of septicæmia in animals, tuberculosis, glanders, some forms of suppurative inflammation, malignant œdema, erysipelas, gonorrhœa and trachoma. In these diseases there is no further chance for dispute. To any one *familiar with the facts* no logical escape seems possible from the conclusion, that they represent a parasitic invasion of the tissues by bacteria. Whenever the method of research is beyond criticism and when the author places his facts fully and plainly before the public, as has been done in these cases, we can no longer question, whether these are facts, we can only impeach the observer's veracity. Less satisfactory is our knowledge regarding human pyæmia, relapsing fever and leprosy. Sufficient evidence has accumulated to prove, that certain parasites are invariably present in those diseases. In the present state of our knowledge the supposition, that these parasites cause those diseases is the most plausible one, but it is not yet a demonstrated certainty. Typhoid fever and pneumonia belong, perhaps, to the same class, but the evidence bearing on them is not yet so extensive. In very many other instances occasional observations have been made, which at least suggest further research in that direction. In these lectures I have not presented every isolated observation scattered throughout the literature, nor have I taken account of some few researches, which bear altogether too much the stamp of unreliability.

What has been done up to the present time repre-

14

sents only the foundation of the germ theory. We
have scarcely progressed beyond the certainty, that
various diseases are really due to bacterial invasion of
the body. Next in order should be the investigation
into the life-history of each parasite. In each
instance it is to be learned, whether the virus multiplies only in the body of the victim, or whether it
can also lead a non-parasitic life under the conditions
occurring in nature. It is to be determined further
on, in what manner the virus escapes from the body of
the patient, how it becomes diffused throughout the
world, and through what channels it enters the system
of the fresh victim. All these investigations seem
comparatively easy with our means and methods. It
is only the knowledge gained by such systematic work,
that will enable us to limit the dissemination of vegetable parasites and to protect ourselves against their
attacks.

More incomplete even is our information regarding
the nature of the struggle between the parasitic
invaders and the animal cells. We are not certain yet
in any one instance, in what manner the vegetation of
the parasites injures the tissues, and we are ignorant
likewise of the mode by which the tissues resist the
invasion. We know only the anatomical appearances,
which indicate in some cases, that the inflammatory
response of the tissues is the mode of self-protection.
For instance, the extension of the vegetation of the
micrococci of pus, and of the tubercle-bacilli (at
least in fibrous pneumonia) is hindered by breast-
works, thrown up by the tissues in the form of granu-
lation-tissue. We know also, that in some instances
the parasites perish in the body of the resisting victim. In the skin, in which the erysipelatous inflammation has passed its height, the micrococci have

disappeared; in the center of chronic tubercular processes the bacilli can scarcely be recognized, and in the blood of animals recovering from anthrax the parasites of that disease are found dead. Such dead bacteria appear granular instead of homogeneous and do not take up aniline colors to any extent. But how they are destroyed we do not know.

The study, which promises the greatest immediate benefits to mankind, is that of the nature of the resistance of the tissues to the parasites. An insight into this will probably give us the clue to the immunity against a second invasion of the parasites, which the tissues have just vanquished. For it is only a complete analysis of this process, that will enable us to aid the tissues in their struggle, *i. e.*, to cure the disease, especially since the hope of finding some remedy, which kills bacteria, but is harmless to animal tissues, has never been realized. Whether the artificial production of immunity by vaccination with mitigated parasites will ever become practical in many diseases, can of course not be foretold. It seems puerile at present, to discuss the desirability of such wholesale vaccination, as long as the possibility has not yet been demonstrated.

How far the germ theory of diseases is to extend in the future, can scarcely be foreseen. In all contagious diseases, in all disorders in which the virus can multiply, we cannot but assume the living nature of that virus, be it in the form of bacteria or of other parasites, for we do not know of any non-living matter, that can reproduce its kind. This consideration shows, how untenable is the hypothesis, once put forth by Billroth, that bacteria act but as the carriers of some "morbific virus," which they do not produce themselves. The view, largely promulgated by Beale, that disease germs represent degenerated bioplasm, stray fragments of the animal organization, which—to use a metaphor—have entered upon a life of disorder and are incapable of returning to their former condition of discipline—this ingenious view is after all but the outgrowth of a fertile imagination, not based upon any demonstrated facts. The germ theory is not limited to contagious diseases. After all the contagiousness of a disorder depends upon, whether the parasites are eliminated in such a manner as to become at once disseminated through the air. Indeed there is reason to think that some parasitic diseases cannot be readily transferred from one victim to another. Trichinosis is the type of a parasitic invasion, yet it cannot be transferred by inoculation. It is hence but logical to search for parasites in all diseases, of which the cause is not fully understood. Apart from the parasitic affections it is scarcely possible to point out any disease, the ætiology of which is absolutely settled except instances of poisoning and deformities of a mechanical nature. But it is narrow-minded to think, that the detection of parasites explains everything. The question of predisposition, obscure as it is, cannot be ignored. It shows more sagacity to investigate, why the bacillus tuberculosis does not attack all beings, exposed to it, than to scoff at its significance, because many can resist its attacks. Moreover we are not to forget that the parasites are not the disease, but only its cause. The disease itself is an alteration of the physiological processes, as a response to some unwonted influence. Of course it may and it often does happen, that the reaction of the tissues is the same to different forms of irritation, be they living parasites or other agencies. Hence a symptom or a lesion may by itself not always have the same mode of origin in different instances.

Bacteria are not the only parasites of the animal
body. Apart from the animal parasites, of more
importance perhaps in tropical climates, instances have
been observed in which higher fungi vegetate in the
animal system. But this is a much less common
occurrence than bacterial invasion. Not only are such
fungoid growths found in the skin on mucous surfaces,
and occasionally in the meatus of the ear, but instances have also been reported of parasitic fungi in
internal organs, especially the lungs. In birds indeed
this seems to be quite a common occurrence,* while
the diseases of insects have all been traced to such
parasitic fungi. But quite a number of observations
on man are also scattered throughout pathological
literature.

Some twelve years ago Grohe and Block observed
the growth of mould-fungi with death of the animals,
on injecting spores into the circulation. This experiment could not be repeated by various observers, until
Grawitz† claimed to have transformed the common
harmless mould-fungi into virulent parasites by adapt-
ing them gradually to the high temperature and
the conditions of nutrition in an alkaline soil,
occurring in the animal body. Spores thus prepared were injected into the blood-vessels, became
arrested in the capillaries, especially of the kidney and
liver, and germinated there, producing mycelia. The
portions of tissues involved are thereby killed, but
without much inflammatory action. If a sufficient
quantity of spores has been injected the animal dies
in from three to five days; if the quantity was
insufficient the fungi are destroyed and the necrotic

*Compare Bollinger, Ueber d. Pilzkrankheiten niederer u. hoeherer
Thiere. Vortraege im Aerztlichen Verein zu Muenchen, 1880.
†Virchow's Archiv, Vol. 81, p. 355.

spots are absorbed. But it has since been shown by
Gaffky and Koch* and by Lichtheim,† that Grawitz
did not transform harmless fungi into virulent parasites, but that his cultures became vitiated by the
unrecognized entrance of fungi naturally pathogenic
to animals. While the common forms of Penicillium
and Aspergillus glaucus are harmless and cannot be
made dangerous, the Aspergillus fumigatus and A.
flavescens are always pathogenic, because they can
readily vegetate in the animal system. On account of
the favorable influence, which warmth exerts upon
their growth, they are very apt to creep into alleged
pure cultures of other mould-fungi kept warm. Such
instances of fungoid infections are not comparable,
however, to bacterial invasions, since the fungi do not
multiply in the animal body, but simply germinate
and grow up to a certain phase of their development.
Grawitz‡ has attempted to study the question of
immunity in such fungoid infections, for the first non-
fatal infection seemed to protect his animals against a
second injection of larger quantities. But on repeating
these experiments with pure cultures, Loeffler§ could
not confirm Grawitz' statements.

The fungus, however, which has of late attracted
mainly the interest of pathologists, produces a clinical
disorder not unfrequently observed in man and some
domestic animals, viz:

ACTINOMYCOSIS.

This disease in man and its fungus were first
described by Israel.‖ It was further studied by

---

*Mittheilungen aus dem Gesundheitsamte, p. 126.

†Berliner Klinische Wochenschrift, Nos. 9 and 10, 1882.

‡Virchow's Archiv, Vol. 84, p. 87.

§Mittheilungen, etc., p. 181.

Virchow's Archiv, Vol. 74, p. 15, and Vol. 78, p. 421.

Ponfick* and identified by him with the affection, previously described by Bollinger in cattle. It occurs also in swine. Since over thirty cases have been observed in man by German authors within the last four years, it cannot be very rare. Moreover the diagnosis can only be made by microscopic examination and hence it has probably been often overlooked. In man it appears in the form of purulent tumors or abscesses, which may spread both by continuity and by metastasis. It can thus simulate chronic Pyæmia. The germs enter often through carious teeth, or through the tonsils, and the tumors then appear first at the angle of the jaw. This is also their most common site in cattle, but in these animals the disease is apt to remain localized. In man its diffusion through the system can be prevented by timely surgical interference. In other cases the disease began in peripheral parts of the body. Twice it has been observed in the lungs of cows presenting the gross appearances of tuberculosis.† In the scant pus of the tumors yellow granules are seen, which the microscope resolves into a network of matted mycelial filaments, partly straight, partly wavy, and partitioned off by septa. At the periphery of these filaments oval and club-shaped bodies are attached in a striking radiating manner, whence the name radiating fungus or *Actinomyces.* The club-shaped bodies probably represent the conidia, for on cultivation appearances of budding can be observed. Between the filaments numerous small granules are often found, which perhaps are independent micrococci, the presence of which complicates the process. The cultivation of the fungus has not yet suc-

---

*Die Actinomycose. Festschrift, 1881.

†Pflug. Centralblatt f. d. Med. Wiss., No. 14, 1882, and Hink. Centralblatt, No. 46, 1882.

ceeded outside of the body to any satisfactory extent, and hence its botanical position is still undetermined. There can be no doubt, however, as to the causative influence of the parasite on account of its invariable presence in this disease, while it has never been detected under other circumstances. The fungus exists in the interior of the diseased tissues as well as in the pus, apparently eating its way into healthy parts. In one instance Ponfick could trace the growth through the walls of a vein, so that the blood-current could detach fragments which formed emboli in distant parts, explaining thus the occurrence of metastasis. Johne[*] and Ponfick have successfully inoculated calves and have thereby reproduced the characteristic disease. Rabbits and dogs were found insusceptible to it.

Actinomycosis presents a notable instance of the discovery of a disease, hitherto unrecognized, and of the immediate insight into its nature by the use of the microscope for the detection of parasites.

---

*Centralblatt, No. 15, 1881.

INDEX.

www.ingramcontent.com/pod-product-compliance
Lightning Source LLC
Chambersburg PA
CBHW021703210326
41599CB00013B/1499